Chronic Pain Warrior

Practical Help and Everyday Hope for Chronic Pain, Illness, and Injury

Davis K Bain

ISBN: 979-8-218-84529-2

Library of Congress Control Number: 2026907661

Published by D.K. Bain Publishing

Cover Design by Iain Oothoudt

First Edition, 2026

Preface

Disclaimer: Reading this book may be emotionally heavy because it's real, containing accounts of my personal experiences with chronic health challenges. I am not a licensed medical or mental health professional; nothing in this book is intended as medical or psychological advice. Psychological terms such as, but not limited to, "trauma," "PTSD," and "obsessive-compulsive" are used for descriptive purposes and are only used in an observed correlation between the listed symptoms and lived experiences of many who struggle with chronic health conditions. Any formal diagnosis or evaluation must be made by qualified professionals. Readers are responsible for how they apply the contents of this book.

The term "Chronic Pain Warrior" (CPW) is used to refer to anyone experiencing chronic pain, illness, or injury. I chose this term because the fight for life in all forms is a real and everyday battle amidst chronic health issues.

Anyone who faces these challenges everyday is a warrior.

Chronic pain, chronic injury, and chronic illness manifest differently in people's lives. While these chronic health issues are lumped together in this book, there are distinct differences between their lived experiences. The commonality between these, however, is the isolating nature of the struggles. Throughout this book, "chronic pain" references each of these everyday battles.

Introduction

Hey there! My name is Davis and for three years now I've been living with Post-Concussion Syndrome (PCS). These years have been disorienting in a way that I never would have expected—in a way that's almost impossible to explain to anyone who hasn't walked through it themselves. I have experienced loneliness that is almost all-consuming, shame that is overwhelming, as well as anger at both nothing and everything. I have seen loved ones who are trying to help, hurt me immensely. I have been disrespected and ignored by many practitioners. But I have also seen some of the best humanity can offer—love in its truest forms. In all I have been through, I wouldn't trade my lived suffering for the world. There is an adventure, a thrilling daily existence, to living with chronic health conditions. It's strange trying to explain how I think of my suffering. I wouldn't trade it for the world, but I would be healed this instant if possible. I live with an urgency to heal yet an eternal gratitude for what I have been through and the noticeable blessings throughout it all.

My intention with this book is to create a practical resource for the chronic pain community. I hope my story will both encourage my fellow Chronic Pain Warriors and bring light to the invisible struggles we face daily. I hope the advice I give will educate the support network of the Chronic Pain Warrior, away from a feeling of helplessness and toward an understanding of their very important role. Lastly, I hope that the sensitive discussions bring clarity, peace, and healing for all readers.

In all things, I write this book out of love. I know that if I have struggled so much, someone else has too. This resource is what I have wanted–maybe it is for you too. I hope this book promotes family unity, rekindled friendships, and immense peace. Please take what I say with a grain of salt. My experience, like yours, is one of one. If you're reading this book because you're trying to help someone else who is struggling, thank you for your effort. If you're reading this for your own struggles, I am so sorry for what you have to face on a daily basis.

This book is organized into four sections. I see each section as a way to practically help those living with chronic health conditions. PART 1 shares my story and struggles. PART 2 contains practical advice for both Chronic Pain Warriors and their supporters. PART 3 discusses some difficult and sensitive topics related to chronic pain. Finally, PART 4 explores passages from the Bible which may provide wisdom and encouragement to those who have chronic pain. Stick with me through this book and I'm confident you'll find practical help and everyday hope for chronic pain, illness, and injury.

Part 1
My Story

In the depths of my worst days, I realized my primary motivation to carry on and pursue better health. I realized that if I was suffering so terribly, someone else must be too. This person, someone who is also struggling with chronic health conditions, is my primary motivation for writing this book. I am hopeful that my struggles and pain will help this person through theirs. Though I would prefer not to share my experiences in detail, I'm convinced that I must. The stakes are too high and the pain too real to withhold the truth about the daily and unrelenting struggles I've faced as a Chronic Pain Warrior. I share to show others that they are not alone in their fight for daily resilience. Please use discretion with my vulnerable accounts.

Below is a list of the prominent symptoms I've experienced over three years. This will give context for my suffering and approach to treatments. The underlined symptoms have become my everyday baseline:

<u>Brain fog</u>, <u>headache</u>, migraine

<u>Neck pain and soreness</u>

<u>Poor recall</u>, <u>eye fatigue</u>, <u>cognitive fatigue</u>

<u>Sensitivity to light, noise, and heat</u>

<u>Exercise intolerance</u>

<u>Depression</u>, <u>anxiety</u>, obsessive-compulsive patterns

Losing the feeling of hunger/fullness,

Tinnitus, dizziness

Insomnia

Chapter 1
A Day in the Life

The following narrative is a present-tense account of one of the many terrible days I've experienced. In a position of immediate financial need, I felt pressure to work, even though I knew I was not physically able. The only opportunity I had before me was a summer landscaping gig through a family connection. I didn't want to do this job, in fact I dreaded it from the time I decided to accept. I knew it wouldn't go well, but I didn't realize how bad it would actually be.

This account was written one day after these events occurred. It captures the momentary agony of a terrible day but does not show the long-term toll of accumulating experiences like these. While a short chapter could never truly express the pain, trauma, and isolation I felt that day, I hope this glimpse into my life illuminates the multifaceted suffering which comes from chronic pain.

My alarm shrieks at me as I flinch awake, desperate to cancel the disturbance. My head is already aching from a lousy night's sleep as I rub my eyes and try to imagine the day's tasks. How in the world am I going to work again? Every time I've tried to work since the injury, I've felt like the job was actually killing me.

Is there anything different about this job? Will it end up like the rest? What about the new coworkers? Will they try to understand or just ignore me?

My mind starts to feel foggy, slow. My mental clarity is gone; it's hard to even think through the day anymore. Decision paralysis about my morning routine kicks in along with the shame about it being for something so minor.

Should I brush my teeth before I eat or the other way around? Ideally, I'd eat then brush my teeth, but the kitchen is upstairs and that involves multiple trips up and down the stairs. I guess I'll just brush my teeth now. Wait, I haven't even gotten dressed, let alone pack my lunch box. There is still so much to do and I can't even comprehend it all. My chest tightens with anxiety.

Somehow, I have gotten everything prepared and am ready to work. I just need a text from the foreman. Why hasn't he texted yet? What am I supposed to do while I wait? It's been ten minutes and still no text about the plan today. What am I supposed to do? The longer I wait, the more I question if I can even do this, slipping into traumatic memories of past work attempts. I can't begin to process this now, I'm way too tired; I guess I'll just watch TV to escape these feelings.

After thirty minutes of television, I'm more dissociated, anxious, and foggy than before, which is my fault. I really need to stop doing things that hurt me, but I also don't know how. Finally, I get a text with the plan, and now it's time to work.

I feel so much anxiety, excitement, and brain fog on the drive to the job-site that I end up going anxiously numb. My chest is tight with fear but I'm gonna keep jammin' to some music, pretending that I'm healthy for a few minutes.

After two hours of working this new landscaping job, I'm faced with the same symptoms as every other job: brain fog, headache, and a gross feeling throughout my body as if I was sick. I'm beyond tired of feeling terrible all the time. I want to feel good, normal, or even half as good as I used to!

As work progresses on this humid, 90 degree day, my brain starts to feel like a balloon about to pop. The pain is scary, to feel this bad without anyone who understands.

Even though the pain is terrifying, I also need this job. I'm actually out of money and don't know what else to do. Besides, I have felt this way and even worse hundreds of times, and I'm still here... It probably can't get any worse. I can push, I can prove that I won't be dominated by my injury, and I can manifest the income that I need!

Time to stop for lunch after three hours. I can feel a less-than empty tank of energy while opening my drink with 180 mg of caffeine. I'm desperate for anything to make this job work. I need this. Existential thoughts race around my head as I eat–maybe I shouldn't work this job, maybe I should have gone home two hours ago...

These thoughts make my current symptoms worse, I can't handle them right now. I think I'll just zone out and watch instagram reels for thirty minutes instead. I just need this caffeine to set in and the nicotine pouches to block the pain, then I'll be good! The concoction of caffeine, nicotine, and adrenaline carry me through another couple hours of work somehow.

It's been three hours since lunch and I'm going downhill fast! Every time I bend down to pick up or adjust a paver, I almost blackout. My vision doesn't feel right anymore, like I'm tipsy in the worst way. I've lost the fun feeling of working, if there ever was one. I suddenly have no care in the world for my coworkers, strange for a guy like me. I am starting to wonder if I should go home now... I remember that the last time I felt this bad, the worst of symptoms came after I stopped working.

Oh no, I totally should have left four hours ago. What am I doing here? I'm such an idiot, pushing too hard when I knew this would happen eventually. I had no idea it would happen on day one though! I feel gut-wrenching shame and failure telling my coworkers I have to leave early. I hate leaving them with the cleanup and finishing work for today. I just want to be helpful. What is wrong with me that I can't be helpful for once?

On the drive home my mouth sticks open and my head locks back. I breathe slow, empty breaths while my mind goes empty. The throbbing pain intensifies the longer I drive. I want—no, I need—to feel differently than this. I would never give this pain to my worst enemy. How am I going to get by financially? I am literally out of money. We already ran the fundraiser, so that's not really an option. I can't work, and I'm still waiting to hear back about disability benefits. How long does it take to hear back?

I cannot believe the pain is still getting worse! It's been a half hour since leaving, and I can't handle it. What am I going to do now, tomorrow, next week? I am miserable.

Once I'm home, I stumble around putting everything away, shaking with adrenaline like after a car accident. With time to slow down and recover, I start to feel depressed, apathetic about everything. I need to feel different.

After taking a bunch of supplements and laying down, the pounding in my head has only gotten worse! Is it from the supplements? I don't even care at this point, I'm just going to keep laying here. Suddenly nausea attacks me so I sit up quickly only to feel vertigo. After sitting still and drinking a little water, the nausea and vertigo slowly subside.

Staring at my bedroom wall I think: Where did I go wrong that this is my life? Can anyone see how bad this really is? What can I do to get by without work? Without any answers, I guess I'll just go to bed.

Chapter 2
A "Healing" Journey

Thirty minutes after the soccer ball hit my head, I knew something was off. The first symptoms of what would forever change my life were beginning to show themselves. This feeling I had was different from past concussions, which were marked by headaches and emotional flares. No, this was something new. I felt out of it, an inability to think. It was as if my brain ran out of gas. I slowly walked home, staring off into the distance as if in a drunken stupor. I gathered my things and decided to head to class, in denial that I had another concussion.

Training that day wasn't the normal mix of calisthenics and running. This day, a morale day, was filled with games and competition. As a soccer player of eleven years, I was very excited to show off my skills. Halfway through training, the ball was lofted directly toward me. While approaching the airborne ball, I made a split-second decision that has changed my life ever since. I chose to head the ball to my friend instead of fielding it with my chest.

If I am to ignore the obvious consequences of that action even to this day, I really don't regret it. I chose to head it because I hadn't had a concussion in a while and was feeling good. I knew if I headed it right it shouldn't be an issue, and besides, I had done it a thousand times in soccer growing up. At that moment, I played like I was a kid again, enjoying the thrill of the game and forgetting past concussions.

My first diagnosed concussion came at the age of twelve from a nasty head-to-head collision in gym class. I felt very few symptoms but we were cautious and got it checked out anyway. Turns out, it was the first of many concussions.

The following concussions came a lot easier when I was fourteen and then fifteen. Until my senior year of college, I kept getting concussions almost annually. As far as doctor-diagnosed concussions go, I think I've officially had four. Including physical trainers and self-diagnosis though (I knew the symptoms well), I've had a total of ten. Up until this last one in October of 2022, I had made a "full recovery" each time. I got back to a full school load and all extracurriculars within a few weeks. In other words, I had a relatively "normal" life until my injury.

I am a born and raised Minnesotan, living in and around Minneapolis my whole life. Growing up, I was a responsible kid who respected authorities and had high academic promise. I was frequently told about my potential to do great things and I was determined to do just that. While my dream was to attend the Air Force Academy, I joined the local Air Force Reserve Officer Training Corps (ROTC) when my application to the academy was denied. I was ambitious, hard-working, and thoroughly excited about becoming a military officer.

For my first three years in the Air Force ROTC program, I worked my tail off and consistently ranked in the top third of cadets. I took many leadership positions, volunteered my time training first-year cadets, and put in countless five-a.m. wake-ups.

For myself and my incredible peers, all of this was in the pursuit and mutual goal of commissioning as the best future leaders we could be. I was excited about the path I was on, driven for excellence, and taking big steps toward my goals. I was passionate about leadership and saw my future role of being an officer as a necessary one. I was ambitious, realizing I could actually better the lives of those I led.

A few months before my injury, I had learned that I was selected for a slot in the United States Space Force as a Space Operations Officer. I liked the idea of joining the Space Force. I was going to be part of one of the first classes of cadets to enter directly into the new service branch. This would give me plenty of opportunity to work with some of the highest caliber folks in the country and help build the newest branch of our military.

All of this and much more was slowly stripped away from me as my recovery went from two weeks to three, three weeks to six, and six weeks to twelve. I began to panic as time went on, my recovery stagnated, and a medical discharge from ROTC grew ever closer.

Much of my grief around this ominous ROTC discharge was related to my prior knowledge and concern about concussions. I knew how potentially problematic concussions can be, I knew that they can have lasting symptoms, and I had seen first hand what that can be like.

Four years before my injury, my aunt sustained a head injury of her own that resulted in Post-Concussion Syndrome. At the time of my injury, she had been battling bitter pain for four years. I had watched her, during these long years, fight for any quality of life amidst a daily level 8-10 pain experience. It hurt to see someone I deeply love suffer so profoundly. Her suffering brought me a perspective that I would try anything I could to prevent this in my own life.

Long story short, her struggles became my struggles too and my worst fears about concussions were realized. The temporary hope of the initial three weeks began to vanish as the weeks went on and my recovery went stagnant. The first stage in any similar experience is shock—the very real feeling as if I were in a nightmare and just needed to wake up. This time was marked by the undoubting belief that I would be able to get back everything lost; that I would be able to commission and become one of the best officers the military had ever seen. There was nothing that could stop me from believing this. I just had to believe I could get back all of the health I had before. I started looking into treatments that I hoped would take away my symptoms and return me to the great, healthy guy I once was.

At the eight-week mark of my "recovery," I had a follow-up visit with the first doctor I saw. He specialized in sports medicine and was well versed in concussion recovery. He told me that I needed to wait, to give it time, to keep resting. In other words, follow standard concussion protocol. After eight weeks of doing that exact thing, I still felt terrible. I was eating clean, staying hydrated, and sleeping well. I was trying to ease into activities, as they recommended, but I still had debilitating symptoms. What more could I have done?

It was scary to feel somewhat similar to former concussions but distinctly different. It was impossible to explain to anyone, but I was scared. Looking into this doctor's eyes, I faced the choice to either trust this "concussion specialist" or to go a different direction with my treatments. I decided that from then on I would let my experience, research, and results drive my path forward. Soon after, I began my chiropractic journey.

I pursued chiro for a few reasons. First of all, my aunt with PCS (mentioned above) had found the most relief from anything she had tried while seeing this chiropractor. I also knew that he was operating outside of western medicine, and that really excited me. Even in my initial diagnosis and research, I was keenly aware of the insufficient medical care provided to PCS patients in America.

The first treatment felt super odd, but for about three days after each adjustment, I felt genuinely decent. As time went on though, the adjustments only held for about a day, and the only solution was to keep going back to the chiropractor. This was no small expense either, I needed to go more frequently and the treatment was getting less successful with time. After a few months of feeling like I was going insane (doing the same thing over and over again, expecting different results), I left that treatment and decided to try something else. I wanted to go a more objective, science-based route after my negative experience with chiro. Time to see the real pros.

Convinced by the chiropractor that there was something structurally wrong with my neck, I visited two of Minneapolis' top-rated orthopedic clinics. Each had renowned expertise with concussion recovery and musculoskeletal issues. All I wanted was to find a real cause, something that could be seen and proven.

The first clinic took an X-ray and explained that my neck was in great shape. They told me that the neck pain would need to be treated with cortisone shots (a pain blocker) and that the neurological symptoms are likely just from the pain in my neck. They essentially said that every neurological symptom I was experiencing, no matter how debilitating, was a placebo effect from the neck tightness and soreness. They ignored the fact that I had neurological symptoms before any neck pain, and that the neck pain came along with the neurological symptoms. They didn't listen to me and sent me packing, feeling like a fool.

Distraught, I left. I cannot explain how tough it is to be sitting in a patient room being gaslighted about my own health. I knew they were dead wrong, but I didn't have the strength to say anything about it. I wanted to explain my perspective but felt so small and weak in that room, helpless. In time, I got over this feeling and built up enough courage to try again.

Earnestly seeking help, I went to another major orthopedic clinic in the Twin Cities. At this second clinic, I was X-rayed again and given an MRI of the neck area. We were trying to investigate a possible correlation with the neck pain and neurological symptoms. When the MRI came back showing no signs of any damage in the neck, I was prescribed physical therapy and psychotherapy.

The physical therapy initially didn't interest me, but after doing more research into vestibular therapy for concussion treatment, I was intrigued. For me, vestibular therapy involved a series of eye movement and convergence exercises aimed at reducing eye fatigue and increasing overall daily function. The first two weeks of this therapy brought seemingly great results: I was performing better on vestibular tests, my eyes felt more relaxed throughout the day, and I could go to the grocery store without a migraine. As the last 3 weeks of that therapy continued though, I started to feel worse. My best attempt to describe it is that my brain always felt overstimulated in the wrong ways. The vestibular function improvements came with the worsening of other symptoms. My mood was completely dysregulated, I couldn't cognitively focus on anything, and I experienced intense headaches during even mild exercise. All of these are baseline symptoms to some degree but vestibular therapy was making them worse. Upon stopping this treatment, I needed a break to recover and plan for the future.

After a few months, I felt ready for something else. I needed real help. I was at the end of myself. I could barely get through work (Solar Engineering at the time), and it was hurting me immensely. My relationships were falling apart, and I felt so lonely in my struggles. Family gatherings and hanging out with my friends brought pain instead of joy. When I would try to spend time with groups, brain fog and headaches led to early departures and relationships fizzling out. I wasn't getting nearly as much done at my job as when I started. I began to worry about my job security. I needed help.

Using whatever courage I had, I reached out to Mayo Clinic. Mayo is renowned as one of the best hospitals in the world and has built a reputation of working tirelessly until answers are found and treatments are administered. All of their clinicians are on salary, which means they're not incentivized to rush patients through the clinic and make a quick buck. They're paid the same either way, so they are, by their pay structure, incentivized to practice true medicine. Mayo is consistently a place where celebrities and foreign diplomats are sent when they experience health complications. All of this fed into my expectation and created a nervous excitement as I waited many days to finally go in for my consultation.

I felt so weak and defeated by my symptoms that I could barely advocate for myself with doctors. I could hardly bring myself to appointments, not having any real hope of getting better. I was more fueled by a need to have reduced symptoms than a genuine belief I could be healed. My amazing grandparents, with my request, accompanied me down to Rochester and supported me through the journey. The three full days of appointments, imaging, and waiting rooms were exhausting without any real answers until the last day. The climax of my time at Mayo was seeing a sports medicine specialist who looked at all of my test results/imaging and issued a treatment plan in conjunction with the consulting physician.

With the backing of one of the best hospitals in the world and advanced imaging, this is what I remember being told: My brain is healthy and shows no signs of damage, and my neck is in great shape and shows no signs of damage. The doctor went on to say that my neck pain was likely causing cognitive symptoms, and that my symptoms would resolve over time. To me, they were saying that my debilitating symptoms had no root-cause or cure and the only thing I can do is cover it up. I felt that they weren't listening when I told them that this concussion was different from every previous one, that it was unique. They recommended cortisone injections as well as topical pain relievers. Additionally, I was prescribed anti-seizure and anti-depression medications for pain and mood regulation. While discussing these pharmaceuticals, the doctor told me that these medications would relieve the pain and the associated neurological symptoms. The practitioner told me that I was depressed. Though I had some symptoms which could correlate, I knew I wasn't depressed at the time. Finally, I remember the doctor telling me about a rehabilitation center which would use vestibular and physical therapy to aid in my recovery, something I had already tried to no avail.

I had already done research into, and talked with fellow Post-Concussion Syndrome patients about the recommended anti-seizure medication. From what I had read, many reported horrifying effects. My aunt (with PCS) was one of those patients who suffered a bad reaction to it. I knew I wasn't going to go the pharmaceutical route, since most people who have Post-Concussion Syndrome see little benefit and instead have strange side effects.

My concern walking into Mayo was that they would try everything to get to the bottom of my issues but not find anything. Nowhere in my mind did I expect to be pushed out after three days of minimal testing, told that everything looked normal—that I just needed to take pills, go to PT again, block the pain, and wait for things to improve.

I was heartbroken and hurt, hopeless for real help. Mayo has the reputation of being the place where untreatable issues see resolution and healing. They are known for their ability to find answers for difficult cases. All I got was more dismissal and true isolation in my invisible disability. In short, I felt like they were saying "you're wrong, you don't know what you're talking about."

I don't remember feeling as numb to this emotional pain as I was driving home from Mayo. I couldn't handle the grief and disrespect at that moment. I just couldn't. I held onto resentment against those doctors for a long time. Eventually though, I forgave them and all the other practitioners who caused me so much grief.

Because this isn't an autobiography, I'll spare you the details of the following two years of treatments leading up to today–two years of relentlessly trying different treatments which mostly made things worse and never provided lasting relief. The disrespect and dismissal that I felt at Mayo continued through many of the treatments I have since tried.

I think my tally on different treatments is up to sixteen now, rounding onto seventeen in the coming weeks of additional testing. I have tried vestibular rehab, sports medicine, two upper-cervical chiropractors, physical therapy, two psychotherapists, acupuncture/Chinese herbs, fascial tissue massage, red light therapy, PEMF therapy, hyperbaric oxygen therapy, numerous diets, and countless supplements. I have gotten X-Rays, MRI's, bloodwork, VR eye testing, and countless qualitative assessments. I, along with dear friends and family, have spent over $18,000 (sadly small compared to some people) on these treatments. The result of this striving is that I feel today, just like I did a few weeks after the injury back in 2022. The brain fog, headaches, and other symptoms have not changed–if anything they have gotten worse over time. While there is value in ruling things out and narrowing the possibilities, I have felt much grief over the generous financial support of others being spent on unsuccessful treatments. I hate the idea that our large financial investment into my health hasn't paid off, but so far it hasn't.

I now carry a tremendous apprehension toward any medical professional and find it impossible to trust doctors. The passion to find answers has slowly led to apathy. The ambition to try and live a "normal life" has mellowed into a slow-paced and very quiet rhythm. Though working is a great thing, I've observed that I am simply unable to do so until I consistently feel better.

Before I bring this chapter to a close, I must add a caveat that not all of the practitioners treated me poorly and a few were extremely kind. Specifically, I need to highlight a functional neurology clinic that was both actually helpful and immensely therapeutic for me. While many of my symptoms were unaffected from this treatment, the outstanding level of care, patient respect, and genuine interest in my health were nothing short of amazing. I also must note that one of the chiropractors I saw shared this same spirit of excellence in his work, truly caring for me every time I visited the clinic. Finally, an emergency room doctor, who started an alternative medicine clinic on the side, has been so helpful to me. Though we haven't yet found something that works, she has treated me with great kindness and dignity through it all. Her clinic and support are truly an oasis of medical care in a desert of western medicine.

As much as I want to stop talking about me, I feel I must go on. Using my experience as an example, I will now share the secondary and tertiary effects which have come from my chronic health struggles. Most people have somewhat of an understanding of the primary difficulties of chronic health issues, but not much of an understanding of the secondary struggles. I hope to show how the secondary struggles can be just as bad— or even worse—than the symptoms themselves.

Chapter 3
Secondary Effects

I can't put into words all of the suffering that I have faced relating to my injury. I can, however, try to paint a picture of the major challenges to daily living. The areas hit hardest in my life are my relationships, work, rest, and routine tasks. I also feel I should share how chronic suffering can change and develop with time.

1. Relationships

I am no psychologist. I won't even try to systematically break down the facets of relationships, in hopes to explain the reason why my health struggles have strained every relationship in my life. I will simply report what has happened over the last few years.

Each relationship, no matter how close, has been weakened by my struggles with health. Generally, the closer the relationship, the more hurtful it has been in both directions. Some of the most painful relational strain has been with my parents and siblings, who I am very close to. I know that they would stop at nothing to help me if they could; they are desperate to help however they can. With that said, it is extremely difficult to maintain a "normal" relationship amidst chronic pain. The family birthday party becomes a battle against my symptoms, the family dinner becomes a place of deepening isolation, and everyday conversations become a source of immense loneliness and sorrow. When my pain is all I can think about, hearing about minuscule family tensions is infuriating. When I'm struggling to get through the day—when I've lost the capacity for empathy—how can I care about someone else's minor concerns?

This conversational distance, if you will, strains any relationship. Usually, the loved one who is present feels disrespected or guilty for the awkwardness between them. The Chronic Pain Warrior, who can't help but think only of their own struggles, often feels guilty and isolated even further. In the end they either drift apart or fight for the relationship, but either way the damage has been done. This has happened to me in all my relationships. I don't carry shame or anger about this. For who is to blame? Instead, I have reconciled with my loved ones many times, building a healthier relationship with awareness and mutual support. This reconciliation with family and friends has always involved some component of confrontation, discussion, and forgiveness. Any healthy relationship takes both parties to put in the work which is needed. In the lives of those affected by chronic pain, this work I speak of is more difficult and needed more often. This is the awareness that can be so helpful: that things don't have to look like they used to and relationships can be expected to be messier than before a time of chronic pain.

I have been single for the majority of the last three years, which means that I cannot speak to those who are married or in serious relationships. I do, however, know that dating can get really messy amidst chronic pain. For me, I was running from my injury as fast and far as I could. I was going to defy the expectations put on me by my PCS. I was going to lead a normal, successful young adult life and no one could stop me.

I had just gotten an exciting job as a Solar Engineer when I had a blind date with one of the sweetest girls I had ever met. She was beautiful and we had similar values, it felt like we could talk forever. We quickly went on a few dates and defined the relationship. We had a lot of fun together, going on adventuristic dates and talking about anything. Eventually, the defiance of my injury caught up to me. My daily symptom level went from a 6/10 to a 9/10. I started to become dissociated and filled with anxiety. I couldn't handle the rigors of a full-time engineering job, family events, and dating someone while having a debilitating chronic injury. But I had learned from a young age in sports that when things get tough, you just keep pushing—so that's what I did.

I tried to medicate the pain at work with caffeine and pain pills. I tried to forget the pain when I was with her, becoming extremely spontaneous to distract myself. It worked for a while, until a couple of weeks later when I realized that I had begun to resent my job, my family, and her. My job was an immovable object at the time, my family couldn't take the blame, and so I began to resent her secretly. It was nothing that she did, she listened to me and tried very hard to accommodate my health needs. It was me and only me.

Eventually I started to ignore her, and after being confronted, I started to panic. This life that I so desperately wanted was becoming impossible to maintain and serious changes needed to happen. After a weekend of camping with a friend, I broke up with her because I couldn't imagine dating her another day. She was pretty hurt and understandably so. There were very few outside signs of my inner turmoil or any real reason why I broke up with her.

The scariest thing about it all, is that the excitement of my life finally looking like I wanted it to, blinded me to the blaring issues. I desensitized myself to the pain. While I knew I wasn't doing well, I was able to ignore it in the pursuit of the life I wanted. The brain is pretty amazing that way; our pain receptors and body signaling can actually be suppressed to unnoticeable levels. This is what led to the pain of the breakup for both of us. While I take responsibility for her pain, I also blame my injury more than anything. I lacked the presence of mind to be aware of my body. I was consciously making the best decision I could, and it led to much pain. A truly scary reality of my life with chronic health struggles.

2. Work

I vividly remember sitting in the HR office, my boss by my side, crying uncontrollably. I was unsuccessfully trying to utter the words "I can't do this anymore, I need to quit." As I sat there, trying to convey with my eyes the tragedy of my situation, my kind boss explained that I would need to quit. I never told him that's what I was going to do, he just knew me so well. He knew I had tried so hard to make that job work but had been struggling for months.

What led to this moment was six whole months of working full-time as a Solar Project Engineer. The nature of the work was usually alone, behind a computer. I produced solar system designs and construction drawings for commercial rooftop solar systems. You might be thinking, "Why would anyone with Post-Concussion Syndrome work on a computer full time as an engineer?" I was trying to prove my intelligence and good brain function against all odds. I also had a degree in Mechanical Engineering and I was broke. This job seemed like the best option for me at the time.

At the beginning, work was really hard, but everyone says that starting in the workforce after graduating was hard, so I assumed it was normal. As time went on the symptoms got worse, but I was medicating with excess levels of caffeine and ibuprofen. Into months three and four of working there, I began to gain weight at an aggressive pace and started to experience suicidal ideations. At this point I thought it was just an issue I had in my head, similar to "having a tough week." I began to lose control of my emotions and saw them ebb and flow rapidly.

Into months five and six, I dreaded going into work more than anything, but I had grown numb to all emotion at that point. I went in with an empty smile and cheerful attitude every day. I continued to pump out designs at an adequate pace, getting praise from my boss for my good work. I had begun to feel like I was dying—like actually dying in real time. Nothing that used to bring me joy did anymore, and I felt a constant tightness in my chest. I was worried sick about the life I was living. I kept pushing; I needed this job. Everything else in my life felt like it was failing and failing fast, but at least I had my work to cling onto. How could I leave the one thing I was actually doing well at? How could I just quit with no other plans?

As the end of the job unknowingly drew closer, the suicidal ideations began to become vivid pictures in my head. I knew I didn't want to commit suicide, but at the same time it was the only thing I wanted, my greatest temptation. During the final week of my employment, I had consistent suicidal ideations and two whole-body break downs. On Tuesday of that week, I was hit with an anxiety attack and gross feeling throughout my whole body. As a result, I left immediately. The following day, the same thing happened again. Thursday, I set an appointment with HR, planning to quit, and couldn't even utter the words.

I experienced a tremendous amount of shame, guilt, and grief leaving that job with no plans. I had been looking into other positions within the company for months, desperate to find something sustainable. I had also heard from friends and family that quitting without another job lined up was unwise. Quitting in this way wasn't a choice as much as it was a move of desperation. I had nothing after I quit but I had finally realized the negative effects work was causing.

There was a strange peace to starting from rock bottom because I knew it was only up from there, I also knew I wasn't actively hurting myself with work anymore. Symptoms didn't subside right away, and I continued to struggle immensely for about a month. After that, I began to see symptoms slow down, weight gain stop, and mental health improve. After three months of unemployment, I finally felt back to "normal," which is the baseline state of health I still deal with today.

I want to mention as a side note that I am eternally grateful I did not succumb to the very real temptation of suicide. This is a topic I'll address more in PART 3. For right now, I use my testimony about suicidal ideations as a way to convey the severity of what was happening in my body and mind amidst a "normal nine to five."

I will yet again spare you the details of this pattern repeating through my employment attempts, but I will offer an overview. I have tried eight jobs after the injury, each causing painful symptoms and ending abruptly. Two of them I quit in the first couple of days, like working landscaping as I described in the first chapter. In the remaining five jobs, I have tried social work, construction, consulting, wilderness guiding, and working as a barista. All of them have left me miserable, all of them were unsustainable, and all but one led to suicidal ideations. This has sadly become my mark for when to quit. I have lost the ability to gauge if something is hurting me and how much, I believe due to the high baseline symptom levels I experience. I know that if I have an unbearable day within the first week, I'll quit. If I ever have suicidal ideations, I'll quit. Otherwise, it's really hard to gauge my own tolerance levels.

I haven't given up on working and hope that someday I can hold a job that doesn't hurt me. For now though, I have to pursue disability benefits (SSDI). The financial stress of being unable to work is immense. The SSDI application is an extremely long process, which has restrictions on income. Even if I got a job, most salaries would exceed the monthly earning limit, making me ineligible for benefits. It's a tremendously slow and arduous process, making me impatient with waiting. Six months in and I still haven't heard back.

My current hope is to go to grad school for counseling and help Chronic Pain Warriors through the intense mental battle of their struggles, the same goal as this book. My theory is that, even though this job would be hard, I would love it enough to get through the hardships and even thrive. With that said, I don't know if I'd be able to handle the day-to-day life of counseling. Additionally, I carry reservations about how counseling is being applied in many cases.

My struggles may not even compare to others. I'm not a provider or caretaker for anyone. This means I have the freedom to live as a nomad, staying with friends and family until I can sustain myself. Many people have to provide and care for others in addition to themselves amidst chronic health challenges. I can't imagine being a parent through a struggle like mine. I don't know how anyone does it. These people are warriors in the truest sense. I have the utmost respect for Chronic Pain Warrior parents, facing chronic pain and the needs of the family on a daily basis. It's not fair, but so many still do it. No matter the cost, love drives people to incredible feats.

3. Rest

As crystal blue water, struck by the summer sun, gently flowed three feet below me, I felt nothing but a migraine. Pristine lakes flowed into waterfall pools and back into lakes at the magnificent Plitvice (Plit-veet-say) National Park in Croatia. European carp, flourishing in these waters, swam right beneath my feet as I walked the gorgeous and expertly crafted walkways. Gazing upon the stunning scenery, all I could think about was when I'd be able to get some air conditioning and what I'd have for my next meal. I was in intense pain and nothing could be done to help me enjoy this miserable day, only to get through it.

I have always been an enthusiast for the outdoors, especially when water is involved. My favorite vacations have usually been week-long canoeing expeditions into the wilderness of northern Minnesota and Canada. Portaging through long passageways from lake to lake while fishing and adventuring through this wilderness has brought me more joy than any other vacation I have been on. The Boundary Waters Canoe Area has been a place of true rest for me throughout my life but especially from 15-22 years old. All of that to say, this national park in Croatia should have been a place of adventure and rest for me, an unforgettable family adventure to Europe, restoring for the soul.

This day at Plitvice though, I remember as one of the hardest on a trip that was just so challenging. That week in Europe happened to be especially hot and sunny every day. I've become extremely sensitive to direct sunlight and heat since my injury, and this was worsened by my supplement regime at the time. I would have about one hour of tolerance until a terrible migraine and brain fog would set in, leaving me unable to enjoy even the best of the day's meals and activities.

The hardest part of it all is that my family, who I was with on this trip, was having an amazing time. They continually spoke of the unforgettable memories, the amazing sights, and how much of a blessing it was to have the whole family (including me) there. At the time, I felt isolated because all I wanted to do was stay in and rest. This was a once in a lifetime trip and it meant so much to my family to continue traveling together. I felt I didn't have a choice to stay back at the hotel, that I had to suppress symptoms for their sake.

I pushed through the misery and fought as hard as I could to manage the pain, all while hoping the day of traveling home would come sooner. I must state that I did have a few moments that were tolerable and actually enjoyable on this trip. Swimming, good meals, and quiet evenings with the family were all among my top memories. If I look back honestly though, I wish I had never gone. It simply wasn't worth the pain, let alone the money and travel time.

The few things that have been genuinely restful, for me, involve a lot of time alone and complete quiet. One of my favorite things to do during hard times, though not easy, is to go to a silent retreat center and stay in a one-room cabin for a weekend. These weekend stays have given me true rest away from life's noise, allowing restoration for my soul. Only when I have been able to get away like this, have I begun to feel my mind unwind itself and reach somewhat of a peaceful equilibrium. I am confident that rest is possible for anyone, but it involves creativity and courage to find it.

I share my experience to show that adjusting to a life with chronic pain can be extremely difficult. Please observe that the things which usually bring joy and restoration for someone's soul, can suddenly stop doing so. The best of memories for the loved ones of Chronic Pain Warriors can be the worst of times for someone going through it. Learn from my experience that soul-level rest is a lot harder to come by in chronic pain; this is often a reason we feel so anxious and burned out constantly. Where can we go to find rest? A long walk used to bring me so much peace, time to process and make big decisions. Now it brings me brain fog and bodily pain. Trips to the Boundary Waters, which used to restore my soul, have become almost impossible. Being stuck in the middle of the woods with no escape or comfort in the midst of the pain brings no rest anymore. Overall, restorative rest has become near-impossible to find.

4. Routine Tasks

Grocery shopping, laundry, dishes, and cooking are obviously necessary functions of a successful and independent life. These very functions have transitioned from simple tasks to tremendous stressors in my life. Grocery shopping has been the thing I hate the most, likely due to the nature of the bright lights, music, and constant eye-scanning. Walking through the aisles is dizzying for me, let alone trying to think of what I actually need to buy. I need to check my phone for each item because I usually lose functioning memory as soon as I walk through the doors. The bright lights, music, people, and task of buying the items I need creates an overwhelming state of brain fog and migraine that renders me barely able to make it through the ordeal. This weekly task feels to me like climbing a mountain.

Laundry is difficult as well because the worst damage has been done to my short-term memory. If you were to tell me your name, there is almost no chance I would remember it, even after telling me multiple times. When I start a load, even if I set a timer, I will often forget about it until the next day. This creates a tough situation (mildew) for me and my roommates. Even if I remember, looking downward to fold it creates neck strain and a migraine. I don't know why this occurs, only that it does. For these reasons I subconsciously avoid laundry until absolutely necessary.

Dishes and cooking fit into the category of any other home task (yard work, vacuuming, and cleaning), tolerable but still very difficult. When baseline symptoms are at a 6/10, it's difficult to get out of bed and make breakfast. It's hard to do anything really. Remembering to do dishes, tolerating the physical demands of yard work, and the noisiness of vacuuming become much more difficult and emotionally exhausting.

Managing these tasks is doable for me, so long as I am not working or overly busy. When I have worked, these are the first things to go. I often neglected basic hygiene and nutrition for the benefit of convenience. This was a survival move. I couldn't imagine buying groceries with a post-work migraine, so I chose frozen pizza instead. What an interesting paradox... The person who most needs a healthy diet doesn't have the bandwidth for it. Even though it is possible to eat healthy under a time constraint, it takes a tremendous amount of work, education, and habit-building to enact this change.

One other daily task that has gotten very difficult is sleep. The same paradox applies that the person who needs sleep the most struggles to find it. I've had many bouts of insomnia, though not present at all times. I will often lay down for sleep and experience jittery alertness. My heart starts to race, my mind spins, and I can do anything but sleep. Knowing that I need sleep only makes it worse as it builds the anxiety about not being able to sleep. This anxiety then makes me even more alert and the cycle of sleep anxiety persists.

It is jarring when the things which used to be easy, relaxing tasks of the week suddenly aren't. I know I'm in good company with all those who have seen their daily tasks become more difficult as a result of health challenges.

5. Time

Earlier, I spoke of the shock that sets in upon realizing that recovery has stagnated. Gradually, this shock has turned to a cycle between anger, apathy, and confusion in my life. Out of the immense anger toward my pain, I have fought against the injury with treatments and psychoactive substances. I've also felt complete apathy toward my circumstances without motivation to try anything, stuck in a state of numbness. Lacking direction and wisdom about what to do next, I've felt overwhelming and bitter confusion. This mental cycle has been dizzying, an ever-changing state of perspective on my suffering. As time has gone on, my anger, apathy, and confusion have been compounded because of the effects of trauma-like experiences. Remembering what has happened to me before, like trying to work landscaping, only amplifies fear in daily life. The more I suffer, the more dizzying and confusing life becomes for me. I know I'm not the only one to live a similar cycle which compounds over time. I also know that many who suffer from chronic health issues experience traumatic moments in the midst of their many struggles.

I am not qualified to really discuss trauma, in all of the intricacies and expertise it requires. Having done some research though, I'd like to point out an interesting observation. In many cases of trauma recovery, the cause is a horrific moment or series of moments from the past, which are no longer happening. In cases where traumatic events accumulated over time, a diagnosis of Complex-PTSD could be appropriate. C-PTSD generally applies for individuals who sustained prolonged, repeated trauma over the course of months or years.

Severe chronic health conditions present an interesting case for a psychologist because the cause of potential trauma is ongoing, unchanging, and unavoidable. In the case where someone's condition is psychologically traumatizing, there doesn't seem to be a sufficient diagnosis. C-PTSD seems to fit the potential trauma of severe, chronic health conditions but it doesn't specifically account for continuously living within the source of the trauma (daily life for some CPW's). Chronic pain, in the immediate sense, cannot be escaped and so the source cannot be removed. It is uniquely stressful in the everyday suffering associated with it. It is an inescapable, potentially horrific reality for Chronic Pain Warriors.

To put it simply: Living with chronic health issues is extremely difficult mentally, in a way that can get worse over time instead of better. I feel as if the lack of ability to change my circumstances is it's own torture. I don't know if the ultimate source is my injury, doctors, myself, family, or any other factors; I just know that my psychological symptoms and struggles, which have compounded the longer I've been injured, have been debilitating at times. Even worse, there isn't a diagnosis which adequately fits the unique nature of my mental suffering.

Within Chronic Pain Warriors, there is a full spectrum of experiences, from mildly bothersome to severely traumatic. Additionally, there is a spectrum of how these experiences affect people. Some are severely affected and others only mildly affected. I am not trying to diagnose anyone here, simply trying to comment on the unique mental challenges for chronic pain warriors which change over time. Even beyond the mental symptoms of the chronic struggles, life just happens.

With time comes many transitions: moving, vacations, friendship drama, and starting new things. Transitions, for me, have become extremely difficult, as I lack the emotional energy to accept them. In any transition, what was stable is suddenly not. This change affects my mental and physical health as well. Life throws many curveballs over time, and these days, those curveballs seem to get me every time.

I live now in a bubble of protection, one that I've put around myself. While this is mostly healthy, complete protection is no way to live a life. Because of the constant tension between protection and trying to live life to the fullest, I end up cycling between anger, apathy, and confusion. Sometimes, I am anxiously fighting toward recovery with yet another treatment. Other times, I give up trying anything and live day-to-day. I am often helpless to change my suffering, so I try my best to protect myself from dangers.

My trust in medicine has strongly diminished with time. Right after my injury, I had a healthy trust for healthcare professionals and their qualifications; today I shudder at the idea of talking to a doctor about any of it. Employment has also become a painful topic for me. The idea of getting a job has slowly become an impossible fantasy. It seems so unattainable due to all of the immense pain I have experienced. Dating seems impossible too, so I have generally stayed away from it. I am terrified of potentially hurting an amazing woman because of my pain. I don't want to put myself into a circumstance where I could inevitably do so. Socially, I am apprehensive to go to a party, and even more to talk to people about what's actually going on. As time has moved on, painful memories have increased my fear of almost everything.

Chapter 4
Blessings Amidst the Pain

I feel obligated to leave you with some positive aspects of living through this pain. I hope to illuminate how I can feel extremely blessed as I write this. I have seen the amazing generosity of people first hand; generosity from people I would not have expected. I've seen others perform my hardest tasks for me in an attempt to bless me and support me. I have been truly blessed with a free trip to Mexico and Hawaii three times, all of which have come at miserable crossroads in my life and have led to much healing.

I've had friends and family stand by me through the darkest of times, not perfectly but sincerely. I've seen money appear almost out of thin air when I had none, and friends reaching out to encourage me spontaneously. I've grown immensely in my ability to have empathy, allowing me to truly comfort friends when they are hurting. I have seen loved ones sit and pray with me during the darkest of times. So often, when I am at the end of myself, a friend has comforted me in a way I never expected.

Multiple people have gone out of their way to get groceries for me. So many practical needs have been filled, and in turn, I have felt so much love. I have experienced love so deep, it destroys any notion of hopelessness. I have been blessed with a silent retreat center to wrestle through the pain, truly rest, and heal. I've been blessed with three amazing clinics, where I've been treated with remarkable respect and dignity. I have become friends with these practitioners, who have given me free advice whenever I needed it. I've come to see who my real friends are. I know who will be there for me in thick and thin because I have seen it play out in real time. I have deepened relationships with my parents, brothers, and much of my family.

As weird as it sounds, I wouldn't trade any of it for the whole world. I certainly want to be done with all the pain today, but I have started to realize the great fruits produced amidst suffering. Maybe suffering actually can be a cause for joy.

I am still alive! I am extremely grateful for that—it's no small miracle. On top of that, I no longer have suicidal ideations! If I do again, I know how to handle them with people I love and trust wholeheartedly. I am a truly blessed man, even amidst my suffering.

In the course of my treatment attempts, I've had two moments that have intrigued me ever since. Two different therapies offered the potential of a quick, full recovery within the following couple of weeks. This, sadly, was not the case, but my feelings toward the possibility fascinate me to this day. Though I should have been thrilled by the possibility of full healing, I found myself grieving. I couldn't understand this. Why in the world would I feel sad by the possibility of being healed? In reflection though, I've realized that suffering can be a grand adventure in itself. The more I suffer, the more I wonder, how will I get through this one?

The best adventures happen when faced with tremendous challenges and uncertainty. The adventurers don't know how they will get through it, but they embrace the opportunity before them anyway. They strap on their boots and start walking, without a full plan. Just like the cover photo for this book, I often have no idea what's over the hill in front of me. But with my boots strapped, I start walking, embracing the thrill of the unknown.

Every day for a Chronic Pain Warrior is an adventure, a challenge in the truest sense. If my suffering and pain were to be relieved (something I still desperately hope for), daily life wouldn't be nearly as much of a challenge. While I would much prefer to be healed right this instant, I am grateful for the adventure along the way.

Part 2
Practical Advice

Thus far, I have shared my story to prove that Chronic Pain Warriors are not alone in the feeling of drowning through daily life. If you are supporting someone who is suffering similarly, I hope this has put into words some of their painful experiences. I also hope this has shed light on their somewhat confusing behavior on the outside, as well as the need for you in their life. I now hope to share actionable advice which helps clarify your vital role as their loved one.

Chapter 5
Dear Loved Ones: How to Help

THANK YOU, on behalf of those Chronic Pain Warriors in your life, for your care, effort, and support. I am sure it means the world that you care so deeply. I hope you are not overwhelmed with a feeling of helplessness, as I often am with my suffering friends and family. I hope you know that your role is a lot simpler than you might think. This burden is ultimately your loved one's burden to bear, and if you're willing, I'm sure it would mean a lot to them if you offered to help them bear it. I hope you can see that providing real help to your loved one can be extremely simple. Allow me to share with you a few suggestions.

1. Ask about mental health and listen.

You don't need to be a therapist to ask about mental health; you just need to be a loving presence. For Chronic Pain Warriors, mental health struggles are very common. With genuine curiosity, ask general and freeform questions about how they're doing. Let them tell you, in their own words, what they're going through. Listen to what truly burdens them without any bias. Assumptions about their burdens can create a painful disconnect between you and them. You may have an idea what they're struggling with and be able to gauge the degree of their struggles, but let them tell you in their own words about what they're dealing with. Leave assumptions at the door. This is a challenge, it takes patience and respect. If done right though, you will provide a peaceful and safe space to talk about the ugly things under the surface.

For me, these conversations have been healing in the most needed ways. Too often, my worst struggles were with mental health and I felt so alone because I thought I had no one I could trust to share these things with. Asking about their mental health can create a safe space to truly bring others into the pain and eradicate the isolation that too often accompanies mental health battles.

If your loved one is struggling, consider asking if they're thinking of harming themselves. You won't shock them into suicide by asking—in fact, I would guess that they'll appreciate the concern. In the months after my intense suicidal ideations, my brother asked me if I was considering suicide nearly every time we talked. This showed me just how loved I was, how he was rightfully concerned about my mental health, and how he would be there if I ever really needed it. In the lives of Chronic Pain Warriors, struggles with mental health can be even worse than the physical symptoms. As loved ones and members of their support team, mental health should be a priority just as much as physical health.

2. Show love with more than words.

With the amount of empty verbal support your loved one has likely received (especially from practitioners), love should be shown with actions, in addition to words. This doesn't need to be anything grand or crazy; just be on the lookout for ways to help with practical needs. The best way to find this out is to ask them "What is hard for you that I could help with?" or "Is there any way I could bless you today?" Remember and make a list of their hardest tasks and greatest needs. You don't need to solve these things, just have the list available if you're wondering how to help. As you seek to show love in action, remember to respect and maintain the dignity of your suffering loved one. More on this in my fifth recommendation.

Show love by listening. Curiosity is, bar none, your greatest asset in showing love. I have nearly cried (from love and joy) every time someone has asked me to tell them—free form—about what it's like to have PCS. They allowed me to take the time and space to share the intimate details. Let your questions not satisfy your own interests and concerns, but give your loved one the dignity of an open-ended question.

To illustrate this, I will share my two least favorite questions to be asked in a quick, passing conversation: 1. "How are you?" and 2. "How is your head?" I often get asked the first question at gatherings where it is inappropriate to truthfully answer ("I'm absolutely miserable," for example). I usually end up going with "hanging in there" or "I'm alright," even when it's a lie.

The second question is demeaning in most circumstances because I am much more than my injury. This question addresses the asker's desire to see me healthy. But at the end of the day, if I am not healthy, this question isolates me. I know that I am a warrior who has battled every day of the last three years. I have survived despite the odds and struggles. If I only ever get asked how my head is, then I feel reduced to the status of a victim. As if I just need to be healed so my friend can stop their worrying. This ignores the reality of the fight and diminishes the resilience and strength built from the years of perseverance. You can ask about their health and symptoms, just make sure it is in a safe environment and you are willing to listen to their full reply. If you're only seeing them in passing, a safe move is to schedule a phone call or other time to catch up where you can both have the time and space to share. Respect the dignity and strength of your loved one! A warrior is inside that trembling body.

I have learned that people often ask biased questions, toward the answer they want to hear rather than the truth. Many people do this subconsciously, and I can't say I blame them. When someone grows sick with worry about their loved one, they suffer angst over wanting to see the pain relieved. With no apparent changes over a long time, the mind simply cannot take any more worry. So we start to have selective hearing and manifest a story to keep us calm. Someone might be talking about a new treatment they are trying, are excited for, and even seeing good initial results. The loved one might, weeks later, ask, "That treatment is still working well, right? I wish you all the health and happiness in the world!" before the person can even reply. The better question would be: "Could you tell me about that treatment, what have you noticed?" One question assumes that the person is quickly getting better (to reduce their own worry), and the other leaves it up to the individual to reply truthfully.

For this reason, I theorize that it's far better to let the burden of the pain be carried by the one experiencing it. We shouldn't carry silent burdens of worry on their behalf. The last thing your loved one, who is suffering greatly, wants to hear is that you are carrying huge burdens of worry and angst. The best thing to do is trust them to carry the burden themselves. Instead of drowning in sympathetic suffering and worry, stay focused on how you can help. I'm not saying to forgo empathy. Not at all. I am saying that the burden which family and friends should primarily bear are those obtained in real-time support (conversation, providing needs, quietly sitting with them, taking them to do something fun, etc.).

When you approach your loved one with genuine curiosity, respect their privacy. They very well might not want to talk at that time, and that's okay! They likely don't have any issue with you; their situation may just be overwhelming or confusing. Even if they did have an issue with you, trust that they will address it when the time is right.

Vicarious suffering is a very real burden often carried by the loved ones of those who are in deep pain. Essentially, vicarious suffering refers to the real burdens carried by supporters amidst the trials of a loved one. This is often accompanied by a guilty feeling of suffering at all in the midst of someone else's intense pain. Please take care of yourself amidst your care for others. You will be more able to provide the support that someone else needs if you receive the support that you need. Reach out to a friend, counselor, or mentor. Talk about your very real struggles and ask for support where you need it. It is impossible to provide for others something which we, at first, do not have.

Like all things in life, love in action requires a balance. In this case, the balance is leaving unhelpful worry behind so that we can focus on helping with the real needs of our suffering loved ones.

3. Search for fun.

When daily reality is nightmarish and formerly enjoyable things are marked by much pain, having real fun is profoundly therapeutic. This is one of the toughest tasks for a friend or family member to do, to help someone who is in great pain to experience genuine fun. I'd say, like everything else, start by listening. Ask questions about activities and things they enjoy. Pay attention when they have a smile on their face. Stay in touch with them and listen for instances of joyful memories. This will have many benefits! Having fun with people is a great distraction from present circumstances. Persistent health issues are often accompanied by mental health struggles—mainly anxiety and depression. For this reason, if possible, try to distract them from their situation with fun. Helping the person to get away from the endless loop of fear and apathy, even if for a little while, is amazingly beneficial.

In my life this fun has looked different than most other people my age. I have had so much fun playing cards with my grandparents, sitting by a fire with a few friends, and playing certain board games. Oddly enough, I really enjoy playing chess and it usually doesn't exacerbate my symptoms. Friends have taken me out fishing on their boat, made meals for me, and frequently welcomed me into their homes. These have uniquely blessed me through some very dark times in my life, giving me a little room to breathe amidst overbearing suffering. Just as these have been my favorite blessings from others, all Chronic Pain Warriors can be blessed with fun, it just takes creativity and effort.

Practice safe invites—ones without any suggested answer. Open-ended questions are very useful here. As you ask, ensure that the person has complete freedom to say yes or no, to share their honest thoughts about your proposal. This is a soft skill, something that is learned and practiced. As a general guideline, look the person in the eyes, speak calmly, and use phrases like, "What do you think about going to ____ on Friday night?" or "Would you enjoy coming for dinner next week?"

Many activities which may seem fun can be hurtful for your loved one. At any time, be ready to leave or listen to them when they say they don't want to do something. Try to do no harm in your pursuit of therapeutic fun.

Even if your loved one ends up hurt by an activity that you planned, know that this is not your fault. Trying to bless your loved one amidst chronic pain is a victory in itself. Know that they likely appreciate the effort, even if they can't express it amidst the pain.

4. Just sit with them.

You don't need fancy words or solutions. You don't need to fix their struggles. The best thing to do is just sit, be patient, and share space during the toughest of times. Your presence and patient endurance will be more beneficial than words through the darkest moments. When I felt the world around me was crumbling away, I cried every time a loved one just sat with me through it. I generally don't cry much; these days I only cry when experiencing a lot of love. Love has been the only thing to break through my emotional wounds and defense mechanisms. I vividly remember the times when a loved one simply sat with me; I will be forever grateful for these memories. Sitting in silence says "I love you," "I am sorry this is so hard," and "I'm here for you through whatever may come," all without saying a word.

There are often no solutions, and trying to solve unsolvable problems will only cause more pain. Not every day nor every circumstance requires this type of support. On a really tough day though, just being present is likely the best option and a great place to start.

The general guideline for supporting someone is to let them lead. If they're miserable they'll likely appear quiet and shut down, so sit with them in the quiet. If they're confused and need to process things, they'll likely ask existential questions and seek engaging conversations. If they're actually having a good day, they'll likely ask about you or show true interest and care for others. No matter what they're experiencing, meet them where they're ready to engage.

5. Protect the dignity and freedom of your loved one.

Everyone needs dignity, respect, and authority over their own life. Oftentimes people with chronic pain lose the ability to work, enjoy social outings in the same way, or be truly productive. The domain they have over their life shrinks dramatically. When this is the case, doing their dishes for them may seem like a menial task that you want to do, but it may actually reduce their damaged dignity. This is true for many tasks. In an effort to reduce the burden on someone, loved ones often just take over responsibilities of the person who is hurting. This, while well intentioned, can be more harmful than beneficial. The best approach to practically help the day-to-day tasks of a CPW is to simply ask about ways you can support them. Ask about their greatest daily burdens and offer to help in the ways you can/want to. Recall my earlier commentary about how grocery shopping has been one of the toughest things for me since my injury. When others asked generally about ways they could assist me, I told them about grocery shopping and as a result they were able to meet my practical need in an immensely loving way.

I suspect this trend of taking over responsibilities is most common among parents who dearly love their hurting child. While this is an act of sincere love, I make the case that the person who is suffering should keep responsibilities. The routine demands of performing menial tasks is often more helpful than harmful. However, sometimes having minimized responsibilities is the best option for a loved one. Do what is best for your specific case. This principle stands in all situations: Respect the dignity and freedom of your loved one, so they will have the opportunity to grow and heal. Try to build their dignity by showing immense respect for them, what they've been through, and the wisdom they have gained from suffering.

Unless imminent suicidal actions are suspected (in which case you should step in), trust your loved one to do what's right for them. It's very hard to hear from a loved one that they are having a terrible day. Our instinct (in love) is usually to want to take that away. My guidance is instead to let your loved one bear the burden. Try to encourage and love them as much as you can. Offer to take off some of their burden with practical help when you're able to do so.

In all things, I guarantee that the Chronic Pain Warrior in your life wants to be loved. Any creative ways you can come up with to catch them off guard with love should be tried. This will bless them immensely. I cannot imagine a higher call in my life than to help show love to those who need it most. You have been given a tremendous opportunity to do just that.

If you feel helpless toward the suffering of someone you dearly love, you are not alone. This is a natural and valid feeling, even a compassionate one. Know that you can help them through the pain, but you are unable to take it away. It would be best if you could, but this is not how chronic pain works. Your role is to come alongside them and support them as much as you can. Protect their dignity and aim to address practical needs. Sit with them through tough times, and look for opportunities for them to have real fun. Whatever you do, listen with curiosity and let them guide you toward the support which they need. Please don't take their burden upon yourself, and don't entertain apathy for even a second. You are able to help just as you are! Your presence in their life is probably more helpful than you'll ever know.

Quick Recap:

1. Ask about mental health and listen.

2. Show love with more than words.

3. Search for fun.

4. Just sit with them.

5. Protect the dignity and freedom of your loved one.

Chapter 6
Dear Loved Ones:
What to Avoid

Please know that your efforts to help wherever you can are always appreciated. While good intentions are a blessing in and of themselves, the things you say and do may end up hurting the loved one you are so desperate to help. Please know that between doing nothing (apathy, silence, distance) and wrongfully trying to help, I would always choose the latter. I'd rather experience pain from someone who is poorly trying to help, than to get nothing from my loved ones.

With the guidance from the previous chapter as a roadmap for genuine help, I'd make the case that if you're able, you should always try to help. Please don't let fear hold you back! Be courageous, be strong, and put in the effort that the truest love requires. You are not qualified to fix this person (no one is), but you are more than qualified to help them greatly.

Your role as a loved one of someone who is deeply suffering is vitally important. Step into that role with confidence that you can actually make a difference. With that said, I feel I must mention some things to look out for. Think of it like putting up guard rails, showing you how to drive down the road of help without running into the ditch of unintentionally contributing to more suffering. Let's walk through a few ways to avoid hurting your loved ones when trying to help.

1. Don't trigger symptoms.

This sounds simple, but it's really quite a challenge. It requires more than you may think. You must actively listen to your loved one when talking about their symptoms. Learn what causes symptoms and do your best to avoid such things. Write them down, make a list, and don't forget it! As much as you can, don't trigger or worsen their symptoms. In whatever you do, try to do no harm.

Symptoms are bound to happen and may worsen when they are with you for no reason. All you can do is control what you say and do. Again, they may have terrible symptoms when they are with you—please don't take it personally. Your role is to patiently listen, ask questions, and do what you can. If you do this well, you will be a place of refuge for your loved one, a much-appreciated safe haven. Going one step further is to actually help reduce symptoms when they're hurting. This could look like cooking a healthy meal, providing a dark room to lay down in, making them tea, going for a walk with them, or just sitting still and sharing space.

All in all, control what you can and don't fret about what you can't. It would be a tragedy for a supporter to accidentally worsen symptoms and then, dwelling in shame, never try to help again. Perfection is impossible and chronic pain is unpredictable, all anyone asks is that you keep trying to support them well.

2. Don't try to fix them.

I know I've mentioned this already, but I must repeat myself. If your loved one is anything like me, they've had many doctors make lofty promises about full recovery, demanding unwavering trust for "the process." In times when this doesn't pan out and they have to leave the provider, it can contribute to medical trauma. If you're not a doctor, then trying to fix a situation that even a doctor can't figure out will only hurt your loved one. Be mindful of the medical trauma they may already carry.

I must clarify that brainstorming potential treatment options, making plans for moving forward, and helping figure out day-to-day needs are amazing things that family and close friends should be involved in. I'm not saying you should avoid helping them pursue new options. I am only saying that you should not try to fix them. There is a difference. The unhealthy "fix-you" attitude is marked by ego and pride. The one who is giving harmful advice is trying to be the heroic friend who rescued their loved one. I suppose you could call this the "savior complex." Check the ego at the door, humble yourself, and meet them side by side.

It's easy for this savior complex to happen to doctors, therapists, and healthy people when interacting with the hurting. I've had three doctors who have treated me like respectful peers, while the rest demeaned me to a less-than status. They were determined that they would be the one to fix me, ignoring the failing results of their treatments. Experiencing this with doctors has become my new normal. The hardest, though, is with my healthy friends. Friends who've been blessed with good health, who have some knowledge of healthy living, can be very hurtful if they don't exercise humility.

I have observed health being viewed in a capitalistic, currency status. I've seen it in myself and many others. With this perspective, some people have more of it and some have less. Those with more health have earned it, while those with less health deserve it. In this distinctly American system of thought, the one who has been blessed with great health becomes the fixer. The fixer believes they will help their friend reach better health, with genius tips and healthy living principles. After all, what they've been doing is working so well. The proof of their superior knowledge is in the pudding of their great health. This is often subtle, and the fixer often has no idea about their harmful words. I see it most in large gatherings and conversations with limited context. My friends, who I still love dearly, have tried to diagnose me or suggest treatments without proper knowledge. I've often heard the following: "You just need to ______." Or "You should try ____."

The problem is one of humility. Neither health nor money work in this capitalistic way, at least not entirely. This kind of prideful interaction leaves the Chronic Pain Warrior feeling defeated and isolated. The grief of a strained friendship hurts deeply, while the healthy friend gets a dopamine rush from their "amazing advice." There is a time when loved ones can sit down with the CPW and actually help with a treatment plan, but this should be done carefully.

Going to doctors when they are needed is wise and right to do. The same is true for counselors and especially trusted friends. A friend trying to help is an inherently good thing. For the friends, family members, and mentors who are the real supporters at the end of the day, come alongside your loved one. Do this in humility, instead of trying to be their savior. If you are experiencing an abundance of health, remember that you could lose it in an instant. Remember that you are not above your loved one in any way. Remember that they need you as a friend more than they need your advice.

3. Be emotionally careful.

This should be obvious, but I must state it explicitly. First, never push your loved one toward something that could hurt them further. Peer pressure is awful for someone experiencing chronic pain and the accompanying isolation. No matter how much you might want your friend to join you in something, let them decide what's best for them. Trust their answer.

Additionally, don't make jokes about their health condition. Many people have made insensitive jokes about my health in a way that further isolated me. I'd advise to steer clear of jokes. Let the CPW make light of their situation with humor, if they so choose. Don't use their health struggles to your social advantage in any way.

Gossip needs to be avoided to maintain the dignity of the CPW. I define gossip here as the sharing of intimate details without permission. The trust of your loved one must be earned and protected. Whenever they share details of their life, struggles, and questions, treat this information as confidential unless otherwise specified.

I'll offer a theoretical example: My friend Andy tells me that he's been in an all-time low spot in life. He shares that he feels overwhelmed by anxiety, completely stuck, and that his marriage is falling apart. He doesn't know where to go or what to do. In this situation, many people with great intentions would text or call their community to share his struggles and ask for prayer and support. I stand firm in this though: The individual must give consent and be in control over where their personal information is shared. A best practice is to ask something like, "Could I share this with our friend Simon? I know he'll want to support you through this too." After you ask, respect their answer. A caveat for this point is that it is right to bring in support and inform law enforcement, if specific plans to harm oneself or others are in place.

Trusting relationships are key for healing. I have personally seen trust broken within close relationships because information about my struggles was overshared with a broader audience. Respect the CPW to share as they see fit. Respect that they should be the ones who have dominion over where their struggles are shared.

4. Don't be afraid to try and help.

Try to do what you think is best. Your loved one will let you know (verbally or by their reaction) if it's helpful. Learn from your loved one. Avoid triggering symptoms and emotional distress as much as possible. Remember that your role is to be a peer in their suffering. Your job is never to fix them, but to come alongside them in their journey.

Too often, fear holds people back from incredible acts of love. Please have courage when facing the doubts and internal questioning about helping your loved one. Remember that effort carries so much weight of love and blessing, even when things don't go as planned. One prominent example is a family member of mine had me over for dinner. Sadly, because of an unforeseen symptom flareup, I had to leave before we ate. I was miserable and stayed that way the rest of the day. I'm sure she felt bad about this to some degree, even though it wasn't her fault. Despite this, she reached back out again a short time later and invited me for another dinner. I am grateful for this persistence and effort.

Try your best to do no harm, and accept that bad days will still happen no matter what. If you cause worsening symptoms, don't allow shame. Instead, focus on how to avoid such things in the future. Have courage in your efforts to support your loved one. Practically love them wherever you can and you can't go wrong.

Quick Recap:

1. Don't trigger symptoms.

2. Don't try to fix them.

3. Be emotionally careful.

4. Don't be afraid to try and help.

Chapter 7
Dear Chronic Pain Warrior

You have been through so much already, and there may be no apparent end in sight. I grieve heavily as I write this, that even one other person has gone through anything like I have. I want nothing more than to help you as much as I can. This whole book is for you, hopefully inspiring courage and rekindling strength. I hope that my story comforts you, that the advice to your support team equips them to support you well, and that my words equip you to courageously face the challenges in your life. I truly hope you can continue healing (physically and emotionally) with confidence. With that, I feel obligated to offer some advice.

Your situation is as unique to you as mine is to me. You know, better than I do, what you need most. Please turn on your mental filter and ignore any unhelpful advice I give. With all of that said, here are a few things that I wish I had known at the onset of my struggles.

1. Develop selective listening.

If you were leading a large construction project, would you take technical advice from a stock broker? If you were to sail around the world, would you ask for advice from someone who had never sailed? In the same way, why should you take advice about living with chronic pain/injury/illness from people who have no experience with it? The people in your life can be tremendous sources of encouragement and wisdom. I'm very much in favor of maintaining many close relationships no matter the circumstances. I will say, though, that you must develop selective listening when it comes to the counsel of others. You must ignore foolish talk from those who can't understand, while listening closely for good advice and wisdom.

In this, I always ignore cliches. They never paint the full picture and rarely offer any valuable insight. Please trust your ability to discern the difference between good and bad advice. No one knows your story, symptoms, and struggles like you do! Most people just don't get it, and they won't unless they actually experience struggles like you have. Trust your gut and learn to selectively listen. I encourage you to hear everyone out when they have suggestions—they might have something that's very helpful! Even when you know the advice they're giving isn't wise, please maintain the dignity for yourself to kindly listen. This is for your benefit, that you would be able to maintain close relationships with those who don't understand your chronic struggles. Ask for wisdom from people who you know are wise. In this process of selective listening, you will be equipped to apply advice in the most beneficial way for you.

2. Courageously take care of yourself.

In the course of managing your symptoms, relationships, and occupation there are bound to be many conflicts of priority. Additionally, your capacity is a lot lower than it used to be, which leads to a painful adjustment. It takes a long time to know how your body will react in most circumstances. Only time can help you understand your symptoms, allowing you to live without pushing too hard.

This balance—like riding a bike blindfolded—is impossible to do perfectly. It feels unattainable at first, until you start to get the hang of it. The wheels start turning and you start to move. Certain tricks and tips reduce suffering and enable you to do more. You might push too hard here or there and need to correct back to a reasonable level of participation.

Yet, like pedaling with a blindfold, we sometimes run into obstacles at high speeds. It's not your stupidity or lack of foresight that leads to this. It just happens as a result of trying to manage dynamic and debilitating health challenges. You won't always have decent days, understand your symptoms, or be able to behave how others expect. Know this and accept that you may let people down when your symptoms conflict with events and others' expectations.

Examples of this from my life are: leaving important dinners early, suddenly quitting jobs where I am needed, telling others (kindly) to stop talking, and cancelling dates at the last second. This may lead to a strained relationship or even resentment. It also could lead to an excess of unwanted pity, assigning you the identity of a helpless victim. In all of the pain and sorrow that may come from taking care of your basic needs, trust that it is worth it.

I don't think it is selfish to take care of your basic needs before the secondary interests of others. I do believe in considering the interests of others more important than my own—this is how I try to live my life. With that said, there is a massive difference between our basic needs and the interests of others. Here, "interests" translates to one's personal desires and pursuits. In this context it is more about what people are pursuing aside from their personal and basic needs. We must first regard our basic needs, then the interests of others if we choose to live this way.

When you get that gut feeling, your internal wisdom about the need for urgent action, trust it. Quit the job, leave the party, cancel the dinner you're hosting, or drop the class. It will probably be worth it in the end. Doing this will avoid more harm to your already burdened body and mind. There are cases where trauma causes real damage and our defense mechanisms act too strongly. I'm not speaking about trauma wounds or anxiety disorders here; instead, I'm speaking about reasonable judgement to protect oneself at the cost of other's expectations. Listen to your instincts and pay close attention to your needs. If you feel conflicted about a decision, seek trusted and wise counsel. Ideally this person understands your health struggles and has known you for a while. Hopefully this counsel can help you navigate the difficult decisions which you likely face often.

3. Find healthy escapes.

On the worst of days, you will likely need healthy ways of escaping deep pain. This doesn't have to be morally perfect, but if you need an escape anyway, you may as well keep healthy escapes on reserve. You probably know which vices are unhealthy for you. Instead of trying to live without any, I hope you can make a list of healthy and effective escapes.

I understand the burning desire to run as far away from the pain as possible; I still find myself doing this today. I give this advice to me as much as to you. I sometimes find myself staying up far too late watching TV to cope with my immense fear. So often, I feel like I'm losing, that I am trapped in a cycle of poor choices. I hope that we, together, can shift our unhealthy coping mechanisms into effective tools for regulation and healing.

Some examples of unhealthy escapes are: binge watching TV or movies, obsessing about a person or thing, doom scrolling, pornography, gambling, binge eating, and many more. In contrast, some healthy escape options are: going for a walk, calling a friend from out of state, late night drives blasting good music (one of my favorites), voice memo journaling in a parking lot, watching a couple of TV episodes, watching a movie, trying a small workout, going fishing, playing disc golf, cooking fancy new recipes, or simply going to bed early.

It is commonly discussed how coping mechanisms can be unhealthy, but from experience, I would argue that delayed processing of the most complex emotions can be quite healthy. Learning to recognize an ugly emotion and choosing intentionally to deal with that at a later date, when you're better equipped to handle it, is healthy. These healthy escapes I mention are ways of doing just that, initiated by our subconscious.

The human mind is, I state again, quite amazing. We can listen when we crave an escape, perhaps an addiction, and redirect that toward something minimally destructive or beneficial. Stop reading right now and start a list of at least three things you can turn to when you need a healthy vice. When despair comes, try something on the list and see what happens. As the first item on the list, put "call your best friend." You don't even have to mention what you're going through if you aren't ready to process. Just shoot the breeze and enjoy conversation. You could text them proactively and give a heads up about your potential call if you want. Search with curiosity for healthy escapes, and in time, you'll find many.

4. Today, take the next right step.

Viktor Frankl's *Man's Search for Meaning* has been the most impactful book in my life thus far. Frankl, a psychologist, recounts experiences within the concentration camps from his professional perspective. He vividly depicts his unthinkable experiences as a prisoner, as well as the confusing reality of life afterward. The entire book revolves around one point: there is meaning to be found within every life, even amidst suffering.

While I don't believe suffering is inherently meaningful, I also don't believe it's necessarily meaningless. Suffering presents an opportunity like no other—an opportunity for dignity, strength, and love where it doesn't seem possible. A great opportunity for meaningful life amidst suffering which often feels pointless.

I can't imagine how uniquely difficult it is for you. This burden that is yours to bear must be so heavy. Think for a minute, how amazing it is that you have made it this far. Think about the times where it seemed endless and you were helpless to do anything about it. You are still here! You're a Chronic Pain Warrior. Through all of the trials you have faced, you have developed great perseverance and strength, even if all you feel is weakness.

I want to invite you into meaningful suffering. Into the healthiest mindset I have known amidst the tornado of mental agony. You don't know what tomorrow or even an hour from now will bring—all you know is what you have right now. Here is the mindset that I have adopted for my life: Take the next right step.

This necessitates a short-term mentality. I'm not saying to forgo long-term plans or treatment options, not at all. I'm saying to do the best thing you can in the situation you find yourself in now. Take one next step in the best direction you can. The challenges you face are immeasurable, but don't let the long-term worry and anxiety affect your present dignity.

The brave manner in which you bear your suffering is meaningful. Meaning is found in the responsibility you bear amidst the pain. To still love others, serve, and help where you can is to live with heroic dignity. In your one life, walk forward with steady progression, addressing real needs as they come. Pursue long-term treatment options with an excited possibility, but not a dependency. You cannot depend wholeheartedly on other people; this is a recipe for disaster. The next right step one day may be trying a new treatment. Some time later, it may be quitting that very treatment. One day it may be volunteering; another day, it may be quitting the volunteering role.

If you don't know what the next right step is, then I have your next right step: wait until you know the next right step. Talk to friends and family, read books, join support groups, and let the wisdom of others guide your path forward. Whether you are pursuing new treatments, continuing current treatments, or taking a break; I implore you to simplify your cares to that very day. What opportunities does today present? How will you take care of yourself? If something needs to change, what's the next right step? What responsibilities do you bear today? The problems we face are too big to solve alone or right now. We must live in today, taking the right next step. After all, what can we gain from worrying about the future?

5. Learn to live without answers.

Understanding the actual functions of your body and mind is like understanding the bottom of the ocean or the depths of outer space. We have a rough layout of the topography at the ocean floor and have seen a few fish, but only a fool would say that humanity perfectly understands what goes on down there. Outer space is much the same. We have observed planets, moons, stars, and solar systems, yet we have little understanding of their detailed workings. We know nothing about the true bounds of our universe. In the human body, and particularly the nervous system, many professions and practices claim an advanced understanding that could lead to healing. But at the end of the day, every treatment attempt is based on a limited hypothesis of what may be happening and what may help. We can't always know the cause of our symptoms, especially for chronic health conditions. Living without a known cause or an understanding of the underlying issues can be very difficult to bear.

This uncertainty is even more difficult when considering the day-to-day sufferings that come and go freely. The pain, which is so great you would do anything to get rid of it, cannot be fully understood. This pain is often compounded by mental health issues—from the chronic health issues themselves (often the case with gut issues and brain injuries) or from secondary life effects. I imagine that when you feel this unbearable pain, it comes with an existential loneliness too. I imagine you feel hopelessness and desperation to find and fix the root cause.

When I have been in this cycle, what has helped me will likely help you too. Find peace in not knowing. A helpful exercise is to write a letter to your previous self at a time when you felt like you were in the midst of this cycle of hopelessness. Write to yourself when you were in the worst of the pain and despair. Try to comfort and calm your previous self. I'd guess that your letter will be more patient and compassionate than how you think of yourself today. The difficult application is to think of yourself today with the same compassion you have for your previous self.

We've been engrained in a culture that manifests dreams, creates the life that we want, and always finds answers. Please don't get caught up in this culture, but instead find peace in not knowing. You might be in the midst of one of the most painful days of your life, leaving you with two options: 1. You could live in denial and play detective to find the exact root cause. 2. You could accept simply not knowing right now.

Spiraling out of control and needing to find the exact root cause will lead to more despair and isolation. This retracing of your steps, desperate to figure out something that will take it all away, often leads to compounding pain. Instead, you should understand, in the day to day, that you cannot know all the intricacies of your pain. Instead, you should walk upright in it. In other words: courageously face it and live wisely amidst it.

You can ask for help from your support team, use a healthy escape to distract yourself, or journal your jumbled thoughts. You can make peace with the pain and take action, which will likely calm the nervous system instead of jumble it more. You can ask for help in ways you really need it, allowing your support team to participate in your health and healing.

Critical evaluation is beneficial, but you should not do your critical evaluation in the depths of pain and isolation. The clouded judgement, dysregulation, and desperation will lead to unhelpful or even harmful ideas. This could isolate you even more. Critical evaluation is better done when you return to relative stability and can discuss things with medical providers and your support team. To use a surfing analogy, ride the big wave until calm waters greet you again. Jumping off the board in the middle of a gnarly tube will only cause more pain.

Learn to live without immediate answers, being patient to problem solve at a future time. Live courageously in community, let people know your real needs, and don't go through it alone.

6. Live in the freedom of forgiveness.

You are already burdened by health issues which seem or are completely unchangeable. Please live free from additional burdens like bitterness, resentment, and anger. I have already mentioned the relational strain that will inevitably come as a result of chronic pain. I also mentioned the effect of people who will try to "fix you". This pain is very real. For me, it often hurts worse than the actual symptoms. I beg you to forgive, freely and fully. This is for your sake, not theirs. A wise man once told me that staying bitter and holding onto anger toward someone else is like drinking poison and expecting them to die. In fact, holding onto it will ruin you far more than them.

There is absolutely a need for courageous and constructive confrontation. Sharing the harmful effect of your loved one's words or actions is essential for keeping a healthy relationship. First, though, I believe you should forgive. When I confront someone and I've already forgiven them, I am not dependent on their answer or attitude toward me. Our relationship and future interactions are, but I am not.

I will repeat this: the relationship's future is dependent on how they handle the feedback, but I am not dependent on it. Thus, I can live free of guilt when wronged by others. I am free to confront and correct in love, not being dependent on their reaction. Friend, live in the freedom of forgiveness for your sake.

This has been hardest for me with therapists and doctors who have hurt me with their care. It is a multifaceted issue, but it's hard for me to forgive the pride of doctors because I end up paying them for their bad care. Similarly with therapists, I have emotional pain from months of treatment that overly deconstructed structures of stability in my life. I ended up getting worse after some therapy sessions instead of better.

Not only have I been misdiagnosed and mistreated, I've lost so much money in the process. Oftentimes I didn't even know how much I was going to owe until weeks into the treatment. With these very real grievances, I choose to forgive in full. I will remember the wrongs done to me so I can try to avoid them in the future, but I choose to forgive those who have wronged me. From this process, through difficult work, I have freed myself from resentment. I now live in the freedom of forgiveness, adding to the list of the forgiven when I am wronged or disrespected. I invite you, with tremendous courage, to do the same.

7. Make this week a little bit healthier.

James Clear's *Atomic Habits* has widely popularized the idea that small and effective habit building leads to long-term change. There's real, proven science behind this. I encourage you to set a recurring weekly goal of making your routine just a little bit healthier. You know what things could be changed, what could benefit your overall health. Slowly integrate one of these things this week, taking baby steps to implement things that last. Once that choice becomes a habit, you are free to implement something else. To help you brainstorm, here are a few ideas I've found helpful and effective:

- Eat veggies before lunch and dinner (highly recommend reading *Glucose Revolution* by Jessie Inchauspé for some research-based, practical food hacks).
- Go for a quick twenty-minute walk after meals.
- Swap your pastry or cereal breakfast with lean protein and fats (ground beef or soup for me).
- Put the phone to bed an hour before sleeping.
- Set consistent, reasonable times for going to bed and waking up.
- Drink water often.
- Journal something short once per day.
- Each evening, roughly plan out the following day.

You know what can and should be changed in your life. Be slow and reasonable to build it into your routine. Use moderation to avoid burnout and plan a few rewards for yourself along the way. In all you try, have the compassion for yourself that a best friend or loving parent would for you.

8. Use any psychoactive substances in moderation.

Psychoactives (caffeine, alcohol, nicotine, THC, etc.) can be necessary for getting by, but they can also make terrifying symptoms and conditions so much worse. None of these are healthy in large amounts. If you can avoid using any of these, I recommend you do so. Psychoactives have a tendency for mood, energy, and sleep dysregulation. In an already dysregulated body, psychoactives can add a confusing variable to the myriad of symptoms which you likely face. Alcohol is especially dangerous for the gut and brain, which are often symptom-drivers in chronic conditions.

In whatever you choose to do, I pass no judgement whatsoever. I trust that you have done the best you've known how to do at each twist and turn, even if it led to addictions or dependencies. Though you will have to deal with the consequences of your own actions, please have compassion for yourself. Remember how miserable you have been. Remember how you've sought answers and found only more pain. Remember the unfair reality of your suffering compared with your healthier friends. Treat yourself as you would a dear friend who struggles in the same way.

9. Count your blessings.

It is so easy for us to end up catastrophizing, seeing only the worst-case scenario ahead of us. I encourage both of us to count our many blessings! Though we face many trials, I guarantee that we are also blessed. I would even go as far as to say that our suffering has blessings within it, this new and unchosen reality which we must now face. Name and embrace your personal growth, added empathy, and whatever else you have uniquely developed through your trials.

You, better than most, know who your real supporters are. Reflect on all the sacrifices they have made for you, on their love both demonstrated and verbalized. Love them back, actively, when you can! Write appreciation notes, buy them flowers, or cook them a meal. Remember that it is better to give than to receive; you will be blessed as you bless others. Love others when you can. We can't always feel empathy or help in the ways we used to, but look for opportunities and they will come.

If these words seem empty, if you can't feel grateful right now, I get it. I often find myself angry at everything, without a shred of empathy or feeling toward others. If this is you today, I encourage you to get a notebook and start on a new page with "Here are my real burdens right now…" After you have expressed the healthy grief of your real burdens, write the following: "Amidst the pain, I have been blessed. One example is…" Leave this blank until you have something to put down. It could be growth, experiences, small moments, or anything that you hold dear.

What I am proposing isn't the denial of grief. In fact, gratitude is a part of healthy grief. Gratitude is the antidote to the mentioned catastrophizing. It's a weapon against hopeless stagnation, a way to live dangerously in opposition to situational depression. I beg you to try! If not today, then tomorrow. If not this week, then next week. Write them down on sticky notes and put them up all over your house! Whatever you try, choose gratitude when you can. I've been tremendously blessed by my own accounts of blessings when I am in the depths of pain. It's as if someone else, who knows me completely, is gently counseling me toward hope and peace.

In all of these suggestions, trust your gut and embrace anything beneficial while ignoring useless advice. You may feel completely alone due to the isolating nature of pain, but you are not alone in the overall struggle. You are the only one who has to face the truly unique challenges which greet you each morning. Those are your burdens to bear and no one else can. With that said, there are many who feel the hopeless stagnation, isolation, and mental health challenges that come with chronic pain. As much as we need friends and family to support us, we also need each other. When you can be vulnerable about what you're going through, you'll likely be surprised about the similar struggles of someone you never expected.

Your story can inspire many! Let others into the ugly realities of your pain and be honest about it where it's safe to do so. Don't live in isolation; fight against that very real temptation with everything you have. Fight for community and freely forgive those who hurt you. Build healthy habits slowly so they actually last. Take care of yourself first and ignore foolish opinions. Live healthily, as much as you can, and practice gratitude!

Quick Recap:

1. Develop selective listening.

2. Courageously take care of yourself.

3. Find healthy escapes.

4. Today, take the next right step.

5. Learn to live without answers.

6. Live in the freedom of forgiveness.

7. Make this week a little bit healthier.

8. Use any psychoactive substances in moderation.

9. Count your blessings.

Part 3
Chronic Pain
and _______

In the following section, I hope to offer my thoughts on sensitive issues as a prompt to future discussions which are necessary and difficult to have. I have found that money, mental health, psychotherapy, medical treatments, and suicidality have been the most difficult of topics to grapple with and discuss. Because I've previously discussed the difficulties of pursuing medical treatments, I will leave further discussion out of this part. These topics are awkward and oftentimes ever-present on the mind of the Chronic Pain Warrior.

I welcome your honest critique as you read. I hope you know that I offer thoughts and observations from my lived experience. While limited in scope, this experience is extremely valuable. It has the same value as anyone else's lived experience of chronic suffering. These discussions should not only happen in this book though, they should continue in sincere conversations with CPW's and their loved ones. These conversations should address the sensitive and real issues being faced at that current time, whatever they may be. We cannot do it alone. Don't shy away from the awkwardness—lean into it with courage and love, even when it's uncomfortable.

Chapter 8
Money

Living with chronic pain, injury, or illness is uniquely stressful on finances. The high cost of non-insured medical treatments combined with the decreased ability to work is like a one-two knockout punch. Not everyone living with chronic health challenges needs to try treatments which are outside of insurance coverage, nor does every CPW need to stop working. Many of us, however, cannot work typical hours because we cannot "manage" our symptoms to be able to do so. We find ourselves in situations where we must find treatment options to get better. Sadly, these can be very costly. Someone could be thriving with a healthy income one day and be out of work the next. They could be comfortable one day and broke the next. Healthy one day and suffering greatly the next. We cannot know what challenges will meet us, nor can we prevent suffering in our lives.

There can develop a strange connection between money and health. When someone is experiencing unbearable symptoms but lacks the money to try new treatments, what are they to do? Meanwhile, this person may see friends or celebrities trying every treatment because they can afford it. Each time I have seen celebrities, friends, or others with PCS throwing copious amounts of money at treatments which yield good results, it's hard not to be jealous.

Wealth disparity can feel unjust, unfair, and outright wrong. One may ask: "Why? What did I do to deserve this? Couldn't they share a little bit of what they have?" Jealousy and envy are easy to feel here, a slippery slope of self-justification and desire. The product of this combination is usually further isolation, anger, and an utter determination to make money. This is how I typically react at least.

When someone feels kicked down by health issues. robbed of independence and the ability to provide, financial security becomes an irresistible craving. So much so that a person may completely forget what happened at past jobs and strive all the more. The chronic symptoms can be further suppressed, and the consequences of pushing too hard can be more severe. A person who feels this probably wants to spite their pain, to show it who's boss. In my first chapter (a day in the life of trying to work again), this is exactly what happened to me. I felt backed into a corner financially, like I would have to claw my way out inch by inch. In this panic, I started the job and pushed too hard. You probably remember how that went for me.

Being devoid of steady income and the ability to provide is one of the hardest things to come to grips with; harder still is actually running out of money and being broke. This immense stress can make every symptom worse and have a profound effect on the body. It can increase inflammation, worsen pain, and reduce cognitive function. This is why I encourage any supporters of the Chronic Pain Warrior to be generous! If able, please consider giving to your loved one. Ask them about their finances in a non-pressuring way. They may be struggling to get by and overwhelmed by this stress. Getting by financially is so messy as a Chronic Pain Warrior. I don't really know how I've gotten through all of this. Some combination of my income, the support of friends and family, government resources, and workers compensation have left me enough to get by through three years.

I've realized recently that the only thing separating me from homelessness is my friends and family. I have received more blessings than I can count from my support team, who have been generous beyond their means. People who have very little have still given to me, which brings me so much love and gratitude. I'll never forget anyone who has gone out of their way to support me, at their own personal sacrifice. This is love in the truest form. There have been many times where I have been financially helpless, unable to work, unable to pay for treatments, and running out of money. Amidst these difficult times, I had to ask for help from others.

At first I hated even the concept of asking for money, but in time I opened myself up to the reality of the situation. I learned that asking someone to consider helping me wasn't "using them" as much as it was presenting them with an opportunity to fill a legitimate need. So many people have wanted to help me but didn't know how. Honestly, I didn't know how anyone could help me either. Finances present a clear opportunity for the loved one to extend support. In the future, I hope to start a fund dedicated to helping those with chronic pain out of financial corners. I want to give people space to breathe and move, financially speaking. Should I have excess income someday, I want to pass on the blessing that so many have given to me.

I cannot emphasize the financial stresses enough. It's an unbearable weight at times. When treatments are usually not covered by insurance, they can drain finances rapidly. I'm not the only one who has chosen to allocate the next month's gas and grocery money toward an experimental treatment. Many even take on debt in an effort to find some quality of life. I can't blame them either. What if it works? What if that $5,000 treatment is the thing that will finally help? Who can make a "responsible decision" when they are in agony each day and a provider promises relief? Such concerns are completely forgotten and "irresponsible choices" suddenly seem right.

Many who suffer from chronic health conditions are in positions where they need to provide for their loved ones. This is especially true for parents. In these situations, I can only imagine the increased weight of financial stress and the need for somewhat steady income. I can only imagine the moral and practical dilemmas of managing chronic pain amidst providing for others. What is this person to do? How can they provide for the imminent needs of others while taking care of themselves and pursuing treatment options? I'd imagine that this situation is always a messy one, a dynamic dance between basic self care, providing for others, and pursuit of healing. These people who do this dance on a daily and weekly basis are warriors in the truest sense. They ought to be respected and honored rather than pitied. We ought to help these amazing people in whatever ways we can.

If you are in this strenuous situation of balancing chronic pain and financial stress, I am so sorry. The immense weight must be so heavy. I encourage you to think outside the box and to ask for support if you truly need it. It is actually responsible and right to ask for help when you need it. I encourage you to ask many people in order to spread out the load. It's far easier for people to know that you're not dependent on their donations alone; this frees them to give responsibly. Platforms like GoFundMe are great for this. Consider trying it out and invite your closest supporters to help organize it. Try to contact people directly, asking them if you could share the fundraiser information. Keep it personal and brief, simply presenting an opportunity. Know that in your pain, you're not the only one who has felt the compounded suffering from financial instability.

Additionally, there is no shame in honestly applying for government support (In the US: SNAP, cash benefits, housing support, disability benefits, etc.). There is a stigma around these resources, typically that some sort of harmful label is placed on the person who receives them. In the end, this is strictly an individual concern, one that I've felt. I have the choice to either view it as the government labeling me or providing real time support when I actually need it. In other words, if you are in need, applying for assistance presents the government with an opportunity to use tax dollars in a way which they were intended to be used. For me, I choose to swallow my ego and honestly apply, accepting the support which I qualified for.

In conclusion, finances can be very difficult and complicated while living with chronic pain, injury, or illness. If you've been blessed with financial security, please consider giving to those who are in need. I cannot express how grateful I am toward those who have helped me. They have shown me so much love in their sacrifices. It's the love behind the sacrifice that I appreciate more than the money itself. It's not the size of the gift or grandness of the gesture, simply that people are willing to be generous with their resources. Remember that it is better to give than receive. I am confident that you'll be blessed in return for your generosity.

If you are in financial need, please consider asking for help and pursuing all available resources! I share all of this to educate and encourage. I am not asking for money nor am I trying to use this book as a means to raise funds for myself. I share these observations and convictions to lead us all to a better understanding of the needs of others. I hope that many would see love expressed through generosity as I have.

Chapter 9
Mental Health

It should come as no surprise that chronic pain, illness, or injury can severely impact the mental wellbeing of the one who bears it. The often surprising aspect, though, is the multiple modalities in which it does so.

The first way, most obvious to outsiders, is by routinely dealing with the pain and symptoms themselves. When faced with a difficult daily burden, a high baseline of suffering, people experience a lowered capacity to handle outside stress. Because of this, the Chronic Pain Warrior must maintain lower stress levels or face major consequences. They must protect themselves from stressful situations in order to manage their current stress, but this presents another problem. What kind of life is marked by always keeping stress levels low, mitigating risk as much as possible? What life is there in avoiding all potentially stressful situations?

Thus, in the pursuit of living as full of a life as possible, this limit is often exceeded. Everyone's baseline level changes frequently, but imagine that this stress level could be quantified and an average stress level could be attained. Someone who is healthy, with many loving relationships and a great career, would have a lower average stress level. This person would be able to healthily take on difficult tasks, try new things, and take risks when sensible. Let's imagine someone else who's in a stressful marriage with four kids and a boss that drives them crazy. This person will have a much higher average stress. This person will not be able to take big risks, handle new stressors well, or try new things, that is until their life calms down a bit.

These mental cycles are common for everyone. We may take on too much and need to dial it back. We may need to confront a loved one and work toward a better relationship. We may need to find another job. No matter the cause, most issues of high baseline stress resolve with a combination of time, creativity, and effort.

This is not so with chronic health challenges. The baseline stress level is higher than average, and there is often little that can be done about it. No matter the cause or severity of the symptoms, having a higher baseline stress decreases tolerance and elevates anxiety. Anytime this figurative stress limit is surpassed, there are often debilitating symptoms and mental spirals. This concept is commonly understood in the mental health world as the "Window of Tolerance".

First popularized by Dan Siegel in his book *The Developing Mind*, this term describes the range of stress where the nervous system can properly function and respond to life's stressors. In essence, we should try to stay within the tolerance window or face dysregulation. This dysregulation can manifest either as hyperarousal (anxiety, irritation, tension, pain, etc.) or hypoarousal (fatigue, brain fog, dissociation, depression, etc.). The goal of therapy, oftentimes, is to expand this window of tolerance and provide tools to help regulate back to within this window.

This is a difficult task for a Chronic Pain Warrior. High stress within the body affects much more than the actual symptoms of the chronic condition. It affects everything. All of a sudden, a person who has pushed themselves too hard and is outside their window of tolerance may feel a sudden onset of strange symptoms. They may shut down and completely dissociate from the world. They may also feel scared and isolated, as if they are the only one to ever experience such things. These limits are often narrower for a CPW and more often exceeded.

I am terrified when, after three years, I still feel new symptoms when I'm dysregulated. This constant fear of developing symptoms, rooting from the effects of living outside of one's window of tolerance, can become cyclical. This cycle can lead a brain to become stuck in fight or flight, and catastrophize about the future. Catastrophizing (roughly put) is the dark glasses which view the future as the unavoidable, unbearable worst case scenario. That nothing will get better and one is completely stuck in the endless cycle of terrifying symptoms.

I will not try to speak for everyone, because the way our bodies handle stress and burnout is very different. I will say though, that catastrophizing is a typical reaction to consistent and inescapable suffering. Though some people remain mentally resilient amidst tremendous struggles, many of us lose whatever resilience we had and live each day in a state of burnout.

I have observed that the strength to endure suffering well can run out over time. Though suffering does produce perseverance, the journey through suffering can feel like losing. It is a dark place to be alone with confusing new symptoms, spiraling mentally but seeing stability all around oneself. It's best described as feeling invisible. If only others could see what's truly happening on the inside, they would surely stop everything and try to help. But they can't see it and it can hardly be demonstrated.

The dysregulated life, outside of one's tolerance window, is debilitating and confusing. The baseline stress of CPW's is much higher, making burnout and stress-related symptoms far more likely. In other words, many Chronic Pain Warriors live on the edge of their tolerance window—vulnerable to any small stressors which come their way. Thus, chronic pain presents a unique challenge to the mental health of the one experiencing it because, in most cases, it cannot be changed in the short term.

The second way that chronic pain can contribute to mental health issues is through the condition itself. Many chronic health conditions directly or indirectly affect the gut or brain, both of which play key roles in emotional regulation and hormonal balance. Additionally, chronic pain often induces a state of stress in the body, which increases inflammation and disrupts regulatory systems. Another way to put this is that chronic pain vastly impacts the undervalued physiological drivers of mental health.

In the case of concussions, mental health challenges such as depression and anxiety have been established as symptoms and part of the overall diagnosis. This is an example of a physiological change which can cause mental health challenges on its own. Though the mental health struggles of someone with Post-Concussion Syndrome are certainly multi-faceted, they can be ultimately driven by the injury itself.

At first, the idea of mental health issues being caused by physiological changes may cause apprehension, and I get it. A common misconception is that mental health issues are solely caused by situational and psychological factors. Another way to put this, commonly held by insurance companies, is that mental health and medical health are separate issues which should be treated separately. The issue is that this understanding paints with way too broad of a brush. Situational and psychological factors can, and do, cause deep mental suffering. They are not the only causes though. We must have an open mind to the many possible causes of mental health struggles. The more I learn and live it, the more it makes sense to equally look at physiological causes as well as the psychosocial factors which psychotherapy typically looks at. I can confidently say that physiological issues can cause mental health issues. A statement that likely sounds obvious but must be expressed.

In my own case, I've thought of it like an octopus. The head of the octopus is the root cause of my mental health challenges, while the tentacles are the specific mental symptoms. I feel like I run the gamut between different mental health issues weekly, as if a different tentacle grabs a hold of me each time. I've tried to treat each specific symptom flareup in the past, but it seems to only exacerbate others. Even if I finally get one of the tentacles to let go of me, I get wrapped up by another. The mental health symptoms come from my root physical health challenges and are anything but predictable. Even if these mental symptoms come from secondary effects (inability to work, relational stress, diminished tolerance, etc.), they can still be attributed to the root cause of my health condition.

In my case, I cannot find a sufficient diagnosis which properly suits all of my mental health struggles, especially when they come and go with time. If something only lasts for a few days at a time, can it really be diagnosed at all? It has never made sense to me that this ever-changing array of mental health challenges can be a root cause in itself. I've always known that there's a separate root cause. I cannot prove this, but I have known it to the core of my being since my injury.

The head of the octopus (Post-Concussion Syndrome) is almost invisible, hard for other people to see. What's much easier to see are the behavioral changes and mental symptoms which change and move with time. Post-Concussion Syndrome has long been discussed as an invisible injury, where no one can really see the symptoms. I know that my condition is not the only one with this reputation though. I'm not the only one who feels invisible in the pain, displaying many secondary effects of the root cause while the root cause remains invisible.

I won't go on about my own mental struggles, but know that I've lived the confusing reality of ever-changing mental states. Many of us Chronic Pain Warriors have experienced a changing myriad of mental symptoms which ultimately stem from physiological health challenges.

Someday I hope to have a diagnosis which could explain all of my mental instability. To at least have something to point to would be an immense blessing. Post-Concussion Syndrome is a potential explanation, but it is vague and unhelpful for the specific mental challenges I face. "Syndrome" essentially translates to "we see a pattern of symptoms but don't understand why it happens". In my case, mental health challenges are often observed with PCS, but I have found nothing about how to treat these challenges in a targeted way.

The nature of many chronic injuries are similar to PCS, with little information about how to treat the mental symptoms in an effective way. Many are currently living with a vague diagnosis that doesn't really fit the symptoms. So many people suffer tremendously without a proper diagnosis, or even with a misdiagnosis.

No matter the root cause of mental health struggles, the head of the octopus if you will, the ever-changing mental struggles for a CPW can be outright confusing. The role in which physical health challenges directly contribute to mental health needs much further study. For now though, I offer this chapter to better equip us to help those who are suffering deeply, providing an understanding of the multiple tiers of suffering they likely face.

Mental health challenges often accompany the high baseline stress of living with chronic pain. When a person's tolerance window is exceeded, all sorts of mental health struggles and dysregulation may follow. Additionally, many chronic conditions have the capacity to cause mental health struggles, creating a complicated and incredibly difficult task of regulation for Chronic Pain Warriors. Mental challenges, when associated with chronic health issues, cannot be fully understood. Only those who have experienced it can somewhat understand the spectrum of ever-changing mental health challenges that come from a body which is chronically hurting. Knowing this, we can be more patient and loving towards those who are dysregulated, even in times of immense struggle.

Chapter 10
Psychotherapy

Note: In the following chapter, the terms "therapy" and "counseling" are used synonymously to describe the general and current practice of psychotherapy.

I have often asked myself how therapy could best benefit a Chronic Pain Warrior. I've wondered if the high cost of therapy is worth it for CPW's. I've wondered what the best therapeutic technique would be for someone with chronic pain. These questions have no single answers but instead depend on the situation the individual faces and the clinician trying to help. With hesitation, I do believe therapy can be life changing for the better in almost any circumstance. I believe it is worth trying, even with multiple therapists until a good fit is found, if the person can afford it.

Let us remember the octopus metaphor, where the head is the unchanging root cause and the tentacles are the specific mental health struggles that a CPW faces. I know, from personal experience, that the manner in which any therapy is conducted is vitally important. Effective therapy for a CPW would have to account for the uniquely debilitating chronic symptoms the person faces while simultaneously treating the mental health issues. Knowing that human beings are truly integrated in body, mind, and spirit, this is an immense challenge.

Therapy, along with every kind of health intervention, cannot be viewed as an ultimate. Healing ultimately comes from within and each treatment attempt should be viewed as a consultation. The hurting person is consulting about their own health with a clinician who can offer treatments, techniques, wisdom, etc. In this view, attempting therapy is simply the act of consulting about mental health with someone who is trained to offer help. For a Chronic Pain Warrior, the question is whether or not the current mental health struggles warrant the time, money, and emotional toll of therapy. From the alternate perspective, one could ask whether or not the current struggles allow a person to continue doing nothing about them. In other words, can the CPW afford to keep going as-is?

Chronic pain is often a relatively immovable force in someone's life, particularly in the short-term. With a few exceptions, chronic health conditions are not substantially altered with psychotherapy. This presents a disparity of potential between the client with chronic pain and the client without. The therapist has little power or ability to change the chronic health issue, which could be the main burden carried by a client.

One other unique challenge to the therapist when treating chronic pain is the client's potential trauma endured through seemingly mundane and routine events. These types of "ordinary" events can cause long-term distress for CPW's, similar to the potential trauma of working in law enforcement or first response health care. Both medical trauma and complex-PTSD could be appropriate here, depending on the situation. The idea is that the individual who bears chronic pain and suffering could experience regular traumatic events, leading to increased hyper-vigilance and chronic stress responses from the body, similar to those seen in PTSD. Many chronic pain warriors have been diagnosed with PTSD as a result of their health struggles, let alone the potential trauma endured prior to or outside of the person's condition.

Imagine that the last time you went to the grocery store, you suffered a migraine worse than you've ever experienced before. This migraine caused debilitating effects which left you unable to leave the house for a couple days. As a result, you missed a dinner with family from another state, two days of work (including the income from it), and a very important date you've been excited about for quite some time. Not only that but you were in so much pain over these few days that any sort of activity was unbearable apart from sitting in a dark, silent room. In this case, you'd likely try to avoid grocery stores in the future, remembering how badly they affected you last time. Now imagine that every time you've been grocery shopping in the last few years, you got a migraine. Over time, you'd likely develop an aversion not only to grocery stores but all retail stores. You'd likely experience a hyper-vigilant fight or flight response to shopping in general, even just seeing stores as you drive by. This example, though specific and extreme, illustrates how the routine events of normal life can cause trauma-like responses for CPW's.

In reality, the building up of these ordinary experiences and the resulting trauma-like responses in some CPW's happens over a long period of time and with a series of negative outcomes. For me this has happened with doctor appointments, grocery shopping, family dinners, a new job, and many more painful experiences that have led to my trauma-like responses in everyday life.

Bessel van der Kolk's *The Body Keeps the Score* is a fantastic resource for beginning to understand trauma and its effects on the human body. As I explored this book through the lens of understanding my experiences with PCS, I struggled to find a sufficient explanation for my PTSD-like symptoms. I realized that for chronic health conditions, the ordinary events of each day can cause stress responses similar to extreme and point trauma sources. These stress responses which can come from ordinary events can lead to problematic, hyper-vigilant threat elimination which is often unneeded. Instead of trying to first remove oneself from the traumatic source (which is step one in most cases of trauma), the person must learn to live in the inescapable stress sources with a reasonable amount of self-protection. It is a delicate balance that a therapist could help a CPW find.

I believe that if a therapist would come alongside the client, compiling a list of the real triggers and trauma-like situations, the client could learn to regulate amidst their known stressors. A therapist could help to enhance the client's self-protection, preparing them to have agency in real-time to protect themselves from the worst of situations. Additionally, a therapist could provide a client with a tool-belt full of tactics for emotional regulation. This could empower the client to boldly face daily stressors again with confidence in their own self-protection and ability to regulate. It is the misfiring of this protection, inappropriate fight-or-flight responses, that can cause the worst of trauma-related symptoms.

I believe a therapist could help clients learn to live with the debilitating physiological symptoms—developing real strategies for navigating life's challenges amidst their condition. This could look like a calendar-style plan where each day (until the next session) was mapped out with strategies for how the CPW could approach upcoming challenges. It could also be a simple discussion of strategies for certain stressful situations. No matter what it looks like, I believe that this practical and reality-focused approach could help a CPW navigate the immense challenges of daily life.

I know that it is possible for a counselor to help someone with chronic pain to heal emotional wounds, lower stress responses, and develop healthy habits. I know it's possible to help a client who is greatly suffering from a chronic condition to see a real meaning to their life and suffering. This specialty in the mental health of those with chronic conditions is incredibly complex, under-developed, and something I plan to dedicate my career to.

If you are a CPW and are looking for a therapist, I encourage you to look for one who specializes in chronic pain and has experience treating trauma. Ideally, this person has personally experienced chronic pain and will be able to empathize. In whatever you try, trust your gut.

Many people have told me that it takes time to establish a therapeutic relationship, that I should give it at least six sessions before I know if a therapist is a good fit. Personally, I don't believe this. I believe we're more intuitive and our subconscious minds more capable than we give ourselves credit for. Trust your instincts. After you see a new counselor, reflect for a few days and then decide if you'd like to go back. Also, counselors are typically $100+ out of pocket, as a conservative estimate. Six weeks of trying out a new therapist is a $600 endeavor, money that could be gas and groceries for someone who can't work. Be wise and critical, yet courageous in your endeavors with therapy. It could be extremely helpful.

It's time that we critically evaluate counseling as it is today for the specific struggles of Chronic Pain Warriors. While it has amazing potential for real help, it also has notable limitations. I won't tell you, the reader, what to do because choosing to seek help is an individual decision. I will say, though, that there should not be hesitation to pursue help when one has the means to obtain it. Especially for a Chronic Pain Warrior, who feels like they are drowning in the hardships of everyday life, seeking counseling may very well be the next right step. Additionally, reaching out to trusted loved ones while being honest about current trials is often a responsible next step as well.

Many people could provide amazing counsel outside of the traditional counseling framework. Some examples include trusted mentors, religious leaders, and family members. I want to train and equip the supporters of the CPW to better help their loved one. This is one of the main goals of this book. As I move forward, I plan to produce resources and training to help accomplish this. I hope these resources can help families support each other, friends help each other heal, and trusted mentors to provide emotionally-healthy support in times of need. To access these free resources, visit chronicpainwarrior.com.

As a final anecdote, I will once again recommend Viktor Frankl's *Man's Search for Meaning*. I highly recommend the book to everyone. In it, he makes the case for logotherapy because of the strength which comes from finding the meaning of one's life in each situation. The goal of logotherapy is to broaden and expand the individual's view of their life to find meaning outside of it. The theory centralizes around the words of Nietzsche, who stated: "He who has a why to live for can bear almost any how." Perhaps the goal of taking away someone's mental agony could be accomplished by not trying to do that very thing. Perhaps helping a chronic pain client to see meaning amidst the pain is better than addressing the secondary symptoms (the tentacles of the octopus) alone.

I will back this up with personal experience. When I've been stuck ideating suicide, after days and weeks of fighting tooth and nail but losing, I have craved anything to help me make sense of the pain. Often, the worst part of the pain is the lack of control and utter meaninglessness of it all, not the pain itself. In this understanding, I came to the logical conclusion that if I was powerless to change my health and my bitter suffering was meaningless, then I have nothing to live for. In this pit of despair, I was immensely comforted by the words of Frankl, challenging me to find meaning within the suffering that could carry me forward. Frankl also challenged me to see the responsibilities which I, and only I, was uniquely suited to fulfill.

Every trainee joining the US military is challenged to "find their why"—what will help them keep going when times get tough and all feels impossible. I had mine amidst my Air Force training, and I never really struggled to put in the work that was needed, even to excel when trials persisted. Those encountering tremendous battles each day, struggling to know how to get by, need to see meaning in their suffering. They need something that will help them endure with patience and positivity. This meaning is always found outside of oneself, so the therapist can guide the client toward the meaning that is definitively present amidst their suffering. In fact, suffering can have meaning within itself. The therapist can help the client to see meaning amidst and through their bitter pain.

This meaning is different for everyone and is beyond oneself. For me, during the toughest of days, I thought of those suffering similarly. I decided that the meaning of my suffering at those times was to better understand the suffering of others, enabling me to one day effectively help those who struggle with chronic conditions. I thought that if I was going through something so bad, someone else must be too, and they're probably feeling as alone as I am. Whatever the meaning, I encourage all individuals with chronic pain to cultivate what Frankl calls "a will to meaning". That is to say, the pursuit of specific meaning to one's own life, within one's current circumstance.

All in all, I present this chapter as a mixture of my observations and opinions. Know that I am not an expert, not a counselor, and not highly experienced with therapeutic technique. I'm just a guy who's lived it and has an opinion to share. My conclusions come from my limited experience. There are many different types of therapy and many different experiences with each.

Your experience is a better guide for you than mine is. The challenges of chronic pain, relating to therapy, are uniquely difficult. Modern psychotherapeutic practice may be missing the mark for clients with chronic pain. It may benefit from critical evaluation, adaptation, and therapists with personal experience. Existential therapy (also called logotherapy) presents a different view of counseling: not to pursue the direct alleviation of mental symptoms, but instead pursuing meaning amidst life's unavoidable suffering. Perhaps we need to take a closer look at the use of existential therapy for its potential adaptations and applications within chronic-pain focused therapy, where the unavoidable nature of suffering is often felt abundantly.

If counseling has been beneficial for you, then I support it wholeheartedly. If it hasn't, then I'd encourage you to approach it with caution or steer clear for now. I hope that the advice contained within this book can equip friends and family to love and support the Chronic Pain Warrior well. In whatever you do, know that in times of suffering which contain internal accusations of isolation, you don't have to be alone. You may be alone right now but you don't have to stay that way.

Chapter 11
Suicidality

Disclaimer: This chapter discusses suicidality, including personal accounts of suicidal ideations. Please only read this when you are ready for such a discussion. I invite you to stop now and skip over this chapter if you think you should. This is a sensitive issue that has profoundly impacted many. If you are in a crisis or are struggling with thoughts of suicide, please pause and reach out for immediate support by contacting local crisis support or emergency services. In the United States, confidential support is available by calling or texting 988.

I hope this chapter will prompt beneficial discussion and lead you toward a greater understanding than you have right now. I hope this discussion will be insightful, encouraging, and beneficial in guiding the Chronic Pain Warrior toward finding hope and life away from suicidality.

Suicidality is defined as "the risk of suicide, usually indicated by suicidal ideation or intent, especially as evident in the presence of a well-elaborated suicidal plan" (American Psychological Association, 2023). In essence, it describes thoughts and behaviors related to suicide within a spectrum. I recommend that everyone does some personal research into the suicidality spectrum, to develop a framework for the definitions.

I am not an expert on suicidality, nor am I trying to produce a systematic review here. My authority to speak about it comes from my experiences. For me, suicidal ideations were a shameful thing—something I never imagined enduring. My suicidal ideations surprised me in their potency, vividity, and logic. I had never imagined feeling such a way, yet it somehow felt different than I had ever imagined. Please learn from me how strange it all can be, how sudden it can come, and what you can do if you feel it too.

While this book is intended to be more practical than academic, I feel I must begin with a few statistics that are rightfully alarming. I never experienced suicidality until after my injury. This opened my eyes to a potential correlation. Though the data has definite limitations, it is still worth considering:

- Research shows that young adults who have a chronic illness are three times more likely to attempt suicide than their healthy peers [1].
- In an Australian study, people with chronic pain were two to three times more prone to suicidality in the last year than those without. As part of the same study, 65% of those who had attempted suicide in the past year had a history of chronic pain [2].
- A meta-analysis of nineteen different studies found that suicidal ideations had occurred within the last two weeks for one in four chronic pain patients [3].
- A 2019 meta-analysis showed that the risk of suicide doubles after individuals experience a mild Traumatic Brain Injury (concussion) [4].

We can clearly see that chronic pain is associated with an increased risk of suicidality. This data begs us to think about the mental health of those with chronic pain. Even though these conversations are uncomfortable, we need to get serious about suicidality.

In previous chapters, I've shared some of my experiences with suicidal ideations, but I want to intentionally walk through what I've been through and the path to my recovery. The only thing I really have, along with many who have experienced suicidality, is my lived experience. While I've had some recurring suicidal ideations after the events discussed here, my strongest period of ideations happened a little more than a year after my injury. It was in December of 2023, nearing the end of the solar engineering job, when I was deeply contemplating suicide, nearing formal plans. The following descriptions are for this period of time.

With three notable suicides in my extended family, we grew up with immense grief around the topic. To protect my family from repeating this pain, I internally vowed that I would never commit suicide while I was young. Many years later though, things changed dramatically. At the lowest of lows, I remember feeling like I was doomed for eventual suicide—I felt I had no choice.

I will try to illustrate this feeling with a metaphor. Please bear with me and try to visualize. I felt that I was on the (metaphorical) cliff edge of life, looking over it as a curious child would on a hike. Behind me was a mountain so tall, the top could not be seen, yet it was the top I needed to get to for relief and healing. The journey to get there was an impossible climb filled with innumerable threats and guaranteed pain. On this climb were mighty beasts, uncrossable chasms, and raging rivers. By all appearances, even attempting this climb would be worse than death itself. I almost knew that the battle through the climb wouldn't be worth it, that I would only end up in more pain if I even tried. I felt that I would not only die going up the mountain, but that I would die having endured much more pain than I needed to. It felt almost masochistic to go on living any longer.

In this predicament, I started to make peace with dying. Feeling stuck between two terrible options, I felt that jumping off that cliff edge of life seemed to be the best option. Not only that, but it felt like a wind began to build, pushing me toward the cliff's edge. Almost like I had no choice anymore, like I was doomed to suicide and there was nothing that I could do about it. In this analogy, the mountain climb was to keep living in denial like I was—overtaken by the tunnel vision of endless trials. To try climbing the mountain meant that I would keep trying what wasn't working, seeking relief with unsuccessful methods.

I share this metaphor to demonstrate the disordered thinking that can be present amidst deep suffering. This metaphor visualizes the many factors going on and how it felt to go through it. It demonstrates the blinding effects of catastrophizing. It was as if, in all of my pain and isolation, there were blinders around my eyes so I could only see two options—suicide or endless misery. I was alone in these thoughts, not because people were unwilling to help, but because I chose loneliness to "protect" others from myself.

No matter how much I didn't want suicide, it felt both logical and inevitable. I felt that I would live with severe pain in isolation forever, that I would never see relief. I couldn't imagine other possibilities; I simply could not comprehend anything else. Even though it was possible to live with much meaning amidst the pain, be helped by others, or be healed of the pain itself, I could not see such possibilities. I was more tempted toward suicide than anything I had ever experienced before; it was overwhelming.

In the beginning of this storm of suicidal ideation, I wanted to die of natural causes and even prayed for this. I began to put myself in slightly risky situations, as if to tempt fate, but it would not bite. As the days went on (two months) and my heart continued to beat, I grew intolerant of the urgently terrible suffering. As is common when something needs to be changed but isn't, desperation set in.

As the desperation of pain worsened, the passive desire to die prompted active consideration of suicide. I did not entertain the idea consciously, but denied to myself that I was even pondering such a thing. At the very thought of suicide, I flinched and my whole body tightened. I was wretched with shame. How selfish was I to even consider it? Who am I, that I would even be tempted by such a thought? I had decided, subconsciously, that I wouldn't tell anyone about it. Not the worst of the pain, nor the desire to die, nor the suicidal temptation. I knew that I should tell others what was going on but thought it heroic to protect them from such a burden. In love, I tried to spare them from it.

The more I tried to forget though, the more I thought of it. I was bombarded by passive thoughts of different methods to take my life. The scary thing for me is that those thoughts felt like they were coming from beyond me (the wind in the above metaphor). I am not speaking about the desire to die—I could trace that back to a logical progression. I felt and sensed that the vivid images in my mind of suicidal actions were not from me. Yes, I wanted to die, but I did not want to commit suicide.

I know I already said that suicide was the greatest temptation I have ever experienced, but hear me out. I wanted to find a path through the terrain of suffering. I was totally lost inside, but I wanted to put in the work to get better. I wanted freedom and healing—they just seemed impossible. The temptation which felt like it was from outside of me was the loudest voice, telling me to just kill myself now so that the suffering and pain could be avoided.

This is likely confusing to read, but maybe the confusion you have when reading this demonstrates the confusing nature of wrestling with these thoughts. Both are true: I wanted to die more than anything, and I didn't want to die. It seemed that to go on living was to willingly accept purposeless torture. So I suppose that the desire to live was suppressed by the weight of the pain I faced. Combined with my catastrophizing, like it would always be the same as the worst of days, I felt bound to eventual suicide.

One other notable experience within this is the desperate desire for control. I wanted to take fate into my own hands. I felt the hand I had been dealt was too much to bear, and for once I wanted to stop blindly accepting my lot. Instead, I wanted to end my suffering. I suppose, above even the desire to die, I desired the control in which I would carry it out.

If this sounds logical to you, it isn't. I am still confused about it all today. I cannot get my mind around all that was going on, but this gives a decent account of what it was like for me to feel it all. No book or academic review of suicidal behaviors can adequately sum up all that was going on in my case, let alone the variety of other individuals who face it. Having said all of this, there were other significant factors in my case that relate to my chronic pain, work, and life in general.

Traumatic Brain Injury is a documented risk factor for suicide. Thus, one could assume that in the process of the brain being damaged, the body's ability to regulate emotions is diminished. I was also at a job that made my whole life miserable, causing flareups of every symptom I listed in PART 1. I remember hating my job so much because of what it did to me, but feeling stuck. I remember having migraines that were so intense I couldn't actually feel them anymore; I just felt a foggy-numb sensation throughout my body.

At the same time, the chiropractic treatments I was doing led to a terrifying flare-up of what felt like bipolar depression. Additionally, I was eating a terribly unhealthy diet, filled with grease and sugar. I was doing this to cope emotionally with all of the pain. My gut felt as if it was tied in a knot at all times. I had been experiencing anxiety and depression for months. I had been brushed aside and disrespected by so many doctors. I felt so alone because no one knew just how miserable I was.

All of these factors could have individually led to a mental breakdown, but combined, they made for quite the confusing concoction. How I handled it at first made all the difference. In trying to protect my family from the burden of what was actually happening, I sent myself into a negative feedback loop with my own fear and isolation, worsening everything else. I remember not being able to feel love anymore. Like I had been irreparably damaged and was doomed. All of this is to say that there are many possible causes that probably worked together to bring me to my lowest low, some things that make sense and many that don't. My case, like that of anyone else who experiences suicidal ideations, is incredibly complex and impossible to understand in full.

Previously, I had mentioned this "out of myself" source of the darkest thoughts, and I want to offer a potential explanation. I have long believed that we are not just physical creatures but spiritual as well. I've observed that there is objective good and evil, along with deception and blurred lines in between. The thoughts I was having were deceptive in nature, and I could tell they were not from myself. I am confident that I am alive today for a purpose, that I was saved from myself in a sense. I can't really explain how it happened, but on my darkest night–when I truly started to consider taking my own life that very night–I felt the need to reach out for help. For months I confidently hid it from others, but that night I felt a need to reach out for help that I can't fully explain.

I texted a few friends that I was in a rough spot and immediately one of my roommates came downstairs. Upon his praying for me, I was completely relieved of the desire to take my own life. I can't really explain it. I was shocked. This full relief lasted for months, I never even desired suicide until a much later date. It was shortly after this that I quit my engineering job, suddenly seeing clearly how hurtful it was for me. It was as if God cleared the scales over my eyes and allowed me to see things clearly: the need for urgent help, the effects of my job, and a path to start healing.

When the ideations did come back months later, I did the same thing. I reached out to dear friends, prayed with them, and quit the new job I had started. Some dark times did come after this too, but instead of feeling utterly alone, I chose to be fully honest about the ugliest of things with those I trusted. I chose not to suffer alone, figure it out alone, or white-knuckle it by myself. It requires the highest courage to tell someone "I really want to die. I have been ideating suicide and need help." This honesty, though, is the beginning of healing and the foundation of recovery.

As time has moved on and through much work, I have stopped feeling the desire for suicide altogether. Occasionally life will present situations that render me desiring death. I have decided though, that no matter how miserable I get, I will consciously live through it. No matter how hard, I will bear it. I know that my supporters are truly there for me because my struggles have proven this to be true. How else can we know who will be there for us? I may desire death again, I may even be tempted by suicide again, but whatever may come I know what will carry me through.

Much of the desperation which leads to suicidal ideations comes from the seemingly meaningless nature of suffering. If my sufferings are meaningless, then my life is meaningless. If my life is meaningless, why not just end it? I maintain though, that no suffering is meaningless nor is any life meaningless. In fact, a life filled with suffering can be the life with the richest meaning. There is meaning to each day, but the meaning I was craving beyond anything else exists and thrives through deep suffering. I may not see meaning in the pain today, I may not see it in ten years, but I choose to live for the day when I will see it and can run after it as much as I can. I choose to live to see the day of my symptom relief or die naturally while waiting. I choose to use my story and my pain to benefit others.

I wrote this book and shared in great detail because I love you. I have likely never met you and probably won't, but I love you. I want you to learn and be encouraged by my story. You may feel utterly alone now. You may actually be completely alone right now, but you don't have to stay that way. You can and should let others into what you're facing, in all the gritty details.

Sometimes when I have shared, it burdened the other person greatly. In other instances, it made for a messy relationship between us. I learned from these experiences and reconciled the relationships, but I have no regret in sharing what and when I did. I guarantee that people in your life would sacrifice more for you than you'd ever guess, that they truly love you. You don't have to protect others from yourself—you can courageously let them in. You can get through this, becoming even stronger and better equipped for the work set before you. There is benefit to deep trials, even if we're blind to them in the thick of it.

If you feel stuck, choose to wait for the days of joy to return, to see the days of freedom that can come. In the same way that you had no idea something this bad could happen (chronic pain, illness, or injury), you also have no idea what blessings could be in store. What recovery, healing, joy, love, fun, and peace are possible if you only wait to see them? Please consider choosing, as I have, that suicide is not an option for you. Please accept your life, whatever it may bring—both pain and joy, peace and grief. I love you, and you have at least one friend in the fight for daily resilience.

I am so grateful to be living today, something I would have never expected at my worst moments. My pain has been terrible lately. My symptoms have been difficult and immensely isolating. Even so, I am extremely grateful to be alive. I have seen so many blessings come in ways I never expected. Better days are coming, I promise. Right now it may be time to reach out for help and start (or re-start) the healing process.

Again, I am not a professional. I'm just a guy with lived experience. Please consider my words a personal opinion offered in an attempt to bring more clarity and discussion to a difficult topic. There are so many resources available, with people dedicated to help. A great place to start (in the U.S.) is 988lifeline.org. It has resources and support available 24/7. You can call or text 988, or chat on the website. Check out the website even if you aren't in a crisis!

Local crisis response teams (real, local people who are trained to help) can be reached through 911, 988, local healthcare systems, or searching online for your area's resources. While you should avoid calling 911 for non-emergency situations, research the resources available so you'll know where to turn if they are needed.

You can contact me at davis@chronicpainwarrior.com if you would like to share your thoughts about this sensitive topic. Though I am not able to provide crisis support and am not a clinician, I welcome thoughtful discussion. I'm passionate about creating meaningful community around this topic and reducing the isolation.

To reiterate, do not use me as a first point of contact if you find yourself in deep distress. Reach out to a trusted loved one and explain the urgency of your situation. If you feel afraid, or need urgent, professional help, use 988 or your local crisis response team.

Part 4
Faith

Please know that I pass no imposition of beliefs upon you. Wherever you're coming from, I hope this book has been beneficial to you. If, for whatever reason, you are avoiding biblical text, then skip over this chapter. Even if you don't believe in God or have a complicated relationship with Him, I believe this collection of biblical text around the topic of suffering and pain could be a great benefit to you. When my soul has felt far from me, the wonderful words in the Bible have brought me impossible peace. In the midst of the tornado of suicidal ideations, biblical text has calmed the storm and restored contentment.

I would encourage everyone to read the Bible fully through, from beginning to end. I hope in doing so, you can make your own conclusions and understand these wonderful words in context to your own life. Studying the

Bible has changed my view from the limited perspective of God I had growing up to a view of an all-powerful, loving God who knows suffering. Even though He didn't have to, He chose to bear human suffering and acquaint Himself with grief (Isaiah 53:3). The following passages are an incomplete resource, a pointer to the greater wisdom contained within the Bible. I hope they bless you as they have me.

If you haven't studied the Bible yourself or have little experience with Christianity, see the Appendix: "Biblical Context." In this resource, you'll find historical context, definitions, and information relevant to the mentioned Biblical figures.

Chapter 12
Chronic Pain and The Bible

King David opens the Twenty-Second Psalm with: "My God, my God, why have you abandoned me? Why are you so far away when I groan for help? Every day I call to you, my God, but you do not answer. Every night I lift my voice, but I find no relief" (Psalm 22:1-2, New Living Translation [NLT]). I encourage you to read all of Psalm 22 for yourself. It's a beautiful picture of grief in real time, lifting frustration toward God, and expressing the genuine struggle in his heart.

These days, it seems our pseudo-Christian, western culture celebrates productivity, health, and abundance—all things God does not seem to value nearly as much. Instead, we ought to treasure the heart more than anything else–the heart that bears all situations with honesty of feeling. We must observe that David, the man after God's own heart, asks God why He has abandoned him. I'd guess this is as much of an observation as anything else. David likely observed many, if not all, things that were going well in his life crumble and fall away. He observed that God was all-powerful and loving, yet had allowed bitter suffering into his life. He was anxious.

I think that it's in complete righteousness before God for David to propose that God has abandoned him. Before God almighty, David asks why he has been abandoned. This is a faithfulness unknown to those who have not suffered, bringing real grievances to God Himself and waiting for a reply. In the same way and to fulfill this prophetic Psalm, Jesus cries out these very words from verse one as He is on the cross of the Roman oppressors. He was being unjustly murdered for crimes He did not commit. Dying a shameful death, bearing the curse of the cross, and satisfying God's wrath meant for us, He cries out to God about the justice which has been denied Him: "At about three o'clock, Jesus called out with a loud voice, '*Eli, Eli, lema sabachthani?*' which means 'My God, my God, why have you abandoned me?'" (Matthew 27:46, NLT).

We must learn, as David did, to honestly express what we are feeling to God. Suppression, in this case, is unrighteous, while honestly voicing the expressions of the heart to God is righteous. You are free and encouraged to be honest with God, no matter how angry, alone, or confused you may be. Live after God's own heart with your honest lamenting (expressing grief and sorrow). I am not encouraging gossip or making broad-sweeping statements about God, simply inviting us into honest lament.

The descendants of Korah relay a similar, yet unique theme in the Eighty-Eighth Psalm. The entirety of the psalm is a beautiful lament. It can instruct those struggling with chronic health conditions about what to do in the midst of the pain. Look how they convey the pain and isolation, the grief over the life they had which is now lost:

> O LORD, I cry out to you. I will keep on pleading day by day. O LORD, why do you reject me? Why do you turn your face from me? I have been sick and close to death since my youth. I stand helpless and desperate before your terrors. Your fierce anger has overwhelmed me. Your terrors have paralyzed me. They swirl around me like floodwaters all day long. They have engulfed me completely. You have taken away my companions and loved ones. Darkness is my closest friend.
>
> — Psalm 88:13-18, NLT

This is not a popular passage for a western church on a Sunday morning. The idea that God has taken away our companions and loved ones, that God's terrors have paralyzed us, is a lament in the purest form. It is an expression of the deepest grief imaginable, before a God who could take it all away but hasn't. It's an earnest plea for help as much as it is a complaint. The authors know that God is the one who saves, and they are begging Him to help.

We can learn from this psalm to acknowledge the realities of dark moments and respond appropriately. We must be honest about the inner thoughts, the deepest pains of the heart. Our society seems to embrace putting up good appearances, pretending to be okay no matter how "not okay" we are. Perhaps it's the lying, the deception of pretending to be what we aren't, that is the true evil in this case. Perhaps honesty and true expression of the innermost thoughts to God is the beginning of healing and product of inner courage. I pray now that you may learn to be boldly honest, as the writers of these psalms were, with God and others.

Job is likely my favorite book in the Bible. I have found solace amidst the isolation of my pain, in the book of Job. It is a beautiful account of suffering and grief before God. I would encourage you to read it all for yourself. It's a piece meant to be taken in as a whole. With that, I want to provide some insight from Job:

> If only there were a mediator between us, someone who could bring us together. The mediator could make God stop beating me, and I would no longer live in terror of his punishment. Then I could speak to him without fear, but I cannot do that in my own strength.

> — Job 9:33-35, NLT

Even though Job seems to be innocent and claims innocence, he fears approaching the Lord. Thus, he will not challenge God directly but instead laments that he does not have a mediator between him and God. He longs for someone to represent him in court with God, as if he has a case against God for cruel and unusual punishment. A statement in 1 Timothy gives us some good news: "There is one God and Mediator who can reconcile God and humanity–the man Christ Jesus. He gave his life to purchase freedom for everyone" (1 Timothy 2:5, NLT). Even when we aren't innocent as Job seemed to be, we can take solace in two truths: 1. Jesus has purchased our freedom! 2. Jesus is a mediator between God and us. If we truly think about God giving His only son to be fully man and yet fully God, what better mediator is there? To know and experience human suffering, betrayal, and denied justice without a shred of wickedness in Himself is an act of true love. Not only do we have a mediator with God in the heavenly courts, as Job longed for, but this mediator loves us.

We have a mediator! This means we can approach God without fear but instead with confidence. This is really good news! We can approach God boldly with freedom from Christ Jesus. We can approach Him with confidence and full honesty. Remember that anyone who believes in Jesus has been adopted as a child of God (John 1:12). Remember that the Father is full of unfailing love (1 Chronicles 16:34, John 1:14). Approach God boldly and honestly, leave deception and dishonesty behind. In the freedom you now have in Christ, be honest with God about how you feel and what you think, no matter how ugly or unpolished it is. I've observed that what I often need during the hardest times is wisdom, peace, and love. Each of these are ultimately from God.

The Old Testament book of Ecclesiastes contains a breadth of wisdom that can comfort, challenge, and encourage anyone. The book is fairly short at just twelve chapters long. Again, I recommend you read the entire book for yourself, so that the words may comfort you in whatever situation you're in. For now though, I'd like to highlight a couple of verses that have brought comfort to me amidst my pain.

"Enjoy prosperity while you can, but when hard times strike, realize that both come from God. Remember that nothing is certain in this life" (Ecclesiastes 7:14, NLT). I have felt the persistent accusation in my life that something I or my community has done caused all of my pain. I've wondered if my family's diet has caused my problems, if I pushed too hard, or if I should have avoided sports as a kid. I've wondered if the decisions I've made about treatments have led to my persistent symptoms. I have felt immense shame about each decision I have made along the way. This verse, like nothing else, silences my intrusive thoughts. It silences my unneeded shame and unhealthy accusations. It simply tells me that God is on the throne and I am not, that God brings both prosperity and hardship.

In Job 1:21 (NLT), it says "The LORD gave me what I had, and the LORD has taken it away. Praise the name of the

LORD!" Thus, it is the Lord who gives the blessings in our life and the Lord who takes them away. I do not decide my own fate nor do I know what will happen tomorrow. I do know, however, that this same God who has taken my good health from me can give it back. I know that this God loves me dearly. Therefore, my suffering has meaning because God has brought it. Remember that the God who has brought hard times can also bring immense blessings, that prosperity is from Him as well as hardship.

One other thing I have faced is the feeling of not being ready or able to try, being unwilling to keep moving forward until I would be fully healed. I've lived many days apathetically waiting to see my situation change. Ecclesiastes 11:4-5 (NLT) has much to say about this:

> Farmers who wait for perfect weather never plant. If they watch every cloud, they never harvest. Just as you cannot understand the path of the wind or the mystery of a tiny baby growing in its mother's womb, so you cannot understand the activity of God, who does all things.

To paraphrase: Don't wait for the perfect conditions, or even ideal ones, to do the work set before you. Do it when you can. You can't possibly understand God's will or purposes with your life, so keep moving forward. Take the next right step and trust that the God who sees you (Genesis 16:13) is faithful. Whenever you are able, courageously work toward whatever you have the opportunity to do, even if it's the smallest thing.

I know how easy it is to count myself out, but what if there are important tasks that God has for me right now, as I am? What if the same is true for you? All things are possible with God (Genesis 18:14)! When Paul pleads with God three times to take away the thorn in his side, a chronic issue he was facing, here's God's reply: "My grace is all you need. My power works best in weakness" (2 Corinthians 12:9, NLT). The amazing news is that weakness is not a disqualifier in God's eyes but an opportunity for His perfect power to work. In essence, God is telling Paul to keep going, trusting Him in times of weakness. Never forget that God can use you, especially in your weakness.

Lamentations 3 is a chapter that must be taken in context. Thus, you'll want to read the whole book of Lamentations, as well as a resource with historical context. Briefly, the book is written by a prophet (likely Jeremiah) during the time of Jerusalem's fall to the nation of Babylon. This invasion was God bringing justice to His people for their rebellion. God's chosen people, though their punishment was just, cried out fervently for God's mercy. Over five chapters, the author cries out, laments, and holds onto the hope of God's love.

With this context, here are a few passages from Lamentations that could be encouraging: "He has drawn his bow and made me the target for his arrows. He has shot his arrows deep into my heart. My own people laugh at me. All day long they sing their mocking songs. He has filled me with bitterness and given me a bitter cup of sorrow to drink" (Lamentations 3:12-15, NLT). Later, the author says "Peace has been stripped away, and I have forgotten what prosperity is" (Lamentations 3:17, NLT).

These passages highlight three very real troubles that come over those suffering from chronic pain, illness, and injury. First, the author conveys the reality that God has brought this bitter suffering upon him. Second, that his community has made a mockery of him, likely leading to immense isolation. Last, he grieves that there is no longer any peace or prosperity in his life. In other words, he feels he has nothing going for him anymore.

Each of these grievances are often felt by those enduring chronic health challenges. It may be easy, when reading this, to dismiss the significance of these challenges, but please empathize with the author– imagine losing your community, losing peace, losing any prosperity, and knowing God is ultimately in control. That is terrifying for me, terrifying because I have felt it.

So is there any hope? Any reason to keep trying? Does God let us suffer meaninglessly until we die? Let's keep reading. "Yet I still dare to hope when I remember this: The faithful love of the LORD never ends! His mercies never cease" (Lamentations 3:21-22, NLT). Later on, it says, "The LORD is good to those who depend on him, to those who search for him" (Lamentations 3:25, NLT). Finally, in verses 31-33, he says "For no one is abandoned by the Lord forever. Though he brings grief, he also shows compassion because of the greatness of his unfailing love. For he does not enjoy hurting people or causing them sorrow" (Lamentations 3:31-33, NLT).

At the end of the day, the Lord is on the throne and in full control. God is sovereign. He has all authority in heaven and on earth. His power knows no end, and still, His love for us won't fail. He will have mercy on us time and time again because He loves us that much. Even if we actually were abandoned by God (though, in Deuteronomy 31:8 and Matthew 28:20, we see that He will never leave or forsake us), it says that we will not be abandoned forever. Yes, He does bring grief and loss, but He also shows loving compassion. In fact, He does not enjoy hurting us or causing us sorrow. This means we are not just puppets getting tossed around for His amusement. We are still beloved children and these beautiful verses present a path through the pain.

The way, as demonstrated in this chapter of Lamentations, is to state the pain in all of its gritty detail. Let the Lord know your lament, grief, and sorrow in full. Then after we have done that, we can remember, with painstaking effort, the promises of God. We can remember that He is faithful and that He will uphold His promises. Thus, we can cling to Him, as a child clings to a loving father, when we are afraid. We can remember His promises and wait on Him to bring them about.

I'd recommend journaling this lament, grief, and sorrow, seeing the jumbled thoughts hit paper and become logical. If not writing, then try a voice journal or making a visual image (drawing, painting, graphic design) of what you feel. Whatever you choose to do, I pray that you may see God through the pain and that He will guide your path forward.

I take great solace in the fact that God has brought about the hardship I face every day, that the Lord has brought about my health struggles. It brings me so much peace, knowing that God is powerful enough to take it away at any moment, and yet He hasn't thus far. It gives me so much joy to know that God will use this suffering. I pray that God takes away your suffering. If He doesn't do that, I pray that He will fill you with heavenly peace and abundant joy.

I will leave you with a short passage from Romans: "Be happy with those who are happy, and weep with those who weep. Live in harmony with each other. Don't be too proud to enjoy the company of ordinary people. And don't think you know it all!" (Romans 12:15-16). I cannot imagine better guidance for the church about how to love the deeply hurting. Paul, in this case, encourages the reader to weep with those who weep and be happy with those that are happy. That is to say, meet others where they're at. This is not something easy or natural, but something that requires sacrifice.

We must pay the price of temporarily foregoing our own emotions to meet other people where they are—side by side, as a peer. To weep with one who is weeping is empathy in the truest form. This is not saying that we should take their burdens and grief as our own. No, just be with them and share it. Trying to steal a burden is the opposite of helping. Trusting that the hurting person can carry their burdens with a little help is beneficial. At the end of the day though, none of us know it all, and we aren't better than anyone. Let our striving in the church be toward love.

May God bless you, in whatever circumstance He has brought you. Remember His promises, remember His faithfulness and love! Your suffering has meaning—bring your many griefs to God. Dare to have hope in the Lord, remembering His promises. If able, read Job, Ecclesiastes, Lamentations, and many Psalms over the coming weeks. I am so sorry for all of the pain. I love you dearly as a friend, though I may not have met you. If you are not following Jesus but want to, I encourage you to simply talk to God in prayer. Confess the wickedness in your life and ask for His help. Ask God to reveal the mystery of the gospel to you, to teach you about His love for you. Thank Him for the forgiveness and freedom that come from Jesus. Finally, and very importantly, seek a local church or trusted Christian friend for next steps. We cannot do it alone.

"The best adventures happen when faced with tremendous challenges and uncertainty. The adventurers don't know how they will get through it, but they embrace the opportunity before them anyway. They strap on their boots and start walking, without a full plan. Every day for a Chronic Pain Warrior is an adventure, a challenge in the truest sense. If my suffering and pain were to be relieved, daily life wouldn't be nearly as much of an adventure. While I would much prefer to be healed right this instant, I am grateful for the adventure along the way."

Contact

Thank you for reading *Chronic Pain Warrior*! I am beyond humbled that you would spend the time, effort, and resources to finish this book. It is a tremendous honor to be able to share my story in an effort to help others. I hope beyond all else that it has brought you practical help and everyday hope.

However this book may have impacted you, please consider leaving a review. Think of it as a way to help the next person find it. The best platforms to leave a review are Amazon, Goodreads, or emailing me. More than reviewing it, the best thing you can do for this book is to talk about it with others. Share what you learned, how it encouraged you, or changes you've implemented into your life.

If you have feedback you'd like to share with me, please email davis@chronicpainwarrior.com. I welcome discussion, critique, and encouragement openly.

For additional content, blog posts, or to order books, please visit chronicpainwarrior.com.

For wholesale orders, please email davis@chronicpainwarrior.com.

References

[1] University of Waterloo. (2017, August 17). Young people with chronic illness more likely to attempt suicide. *ScienceDaily*. Retrieved September 18, 2025 from www.sciencedaily.com/releases/2017/08/170817110905.htm

[2] Campbell G, Darke S, Bruno R, Degenhardt L. The prevalence and correlates of chronic pain and suicidality in a nationally representative sample. Aust N Z J Psychiatry. 2015 Sep;49(9):803-11. doi: 10.1177/0004867415569795. Epub 2015 Feb 19. PMID: 25698809.

[3] Kwon CY, Lee B. Prevalence of suicidal behavior in patients with chronic pain: a systematic review and meta-analysis of observational studies. Front Psychol. 2023 Sep 29;14:1217299. doi: 10.3389/fpsyg.2023.1217299. PMID: 37842717; PMCID: PMC10576560.

[4] Fralick M, Sy E, Hassan A, Burke MJ, Mostofsky E, Karsies T. Association of Concussion With the Risk of Suicide: A Systematic Review and Meta-analysis. JAMA Neurol. 2019 Feb 1;76(2):144-151. doi: 10.1001/jamaneurol.2018.3487. PMID: 30419085; PMCID: PMC6439954.

Bibliography

Holy Bible

New Living Translation. *Holy Bible*. Wheaton, IL: Tyndale House
Publishers, ©1996, 2004, 2015.

Non-Fiction Books

Clear, James. *Atomic Habits*: An Easy & Proven Way to Build Good
Habits & Break Bad Ones. New York: Avery, 2018.
Frankl, Viktor E. *Man's Search for Meaning*. Boston: Beacon Press,
2006.
Inchauspé, Jessie. *Glucose Revolution*: The Life-Changing Power of
Balancing Your Blood Sugar. New York: Simon & Schuster, 2022.
Siegel, Daniel J. *The Developing Mind*: How Relationships and the
Brain Interact to Shape Who We Are. 3rd ed. New York: Guilford
Press, 2020.
van der Kolk, Bessel. *The Body Keeps the Score: Brain, Mind, and Body
in the Healing of Trauma*. New York: Penguin Books, 2015.

Appendix: Biblical Context

The following terms are used within Chapter 12 - "Chronic Pain and The Bible." Each term is followed by definitions and/or historical context. I am not a theologian or minister; thus, the following definitions are a layman's attempt at necessary context for those who aren't Christian or are new to Christianity. The order is intended to match the order of chapter 12, allowing readers to reference as they read.

Ancient Israel

Ancient Israel is the nation and people whose history, worship, and tribulations form the Hebrew Scriptures (Old Testament). Israel received its name when its ancestor Jacob was renamed "Israel" after wrestling with God; the name translates to "One who wrestles with God".

Jerusalem

Around 930 B.C., the tribe of Judah split from the nation of ancient Israel. Jerusalem was the capital city of Judah in the south, while Samaria was the capital city of Israel in the north.

The Roman Empire

Rome was the political power ruling over Israel during Jesus' lifetime. Crucifixion was a Roman method of execution meant to humiliate and shame the guilty party. The historical man Jesus of Nazareth was crucified. The Israelites thought that the messiah would come in military power to defeat the Romans.

David

An Israelite king around 1000 BC. He famously killed Goliath, a giant warrior from a rival nation who had challenged Israel. David was said to be "a man after God's own heart." This means that God had chosen him to be king because of a likeness between David's heart and God's. In layman's terms, God and David cared deeply about the same things. David often laments due to the many nations and fellow Israelites who seem to want to kill him. At one point, David had to hide from his own son's attempted coup.

Psalms

Within the Bible, there is a book of 150 songs, also called "psalms". These were to be distributed to the nation of Israel and served the purposes of encouragement, comfort, grief, love, and reminding about the truths of God. These Psalms were written by King David (73), Asaph (12), The Descendents of Korah (11), and 54 more by assorted and unknown authors.

Matthew

Matthew is a book of the New Testament, written by Matthew who was a disciple of Jesus. This book is one of four books called "gospels," which are written accounts of the life of Jesus.

The Descendents of Korah

A group of Israelites who were members of the tribe of priests in Israel. Their ancestor (Korah) led a rebellion and was divinely punished for it. Korah's descendents survived; however, and served as worship leaders, song writers, and gatekeepers. They represent an informed perspective of both divine judgement and divine grace.

"Lament"

An expression of grief, loss, or despair. Within the Bible, lament often refers to these expressions being directed to God, with faith that God can help.

Job

A book of the Old Testament which broadly describes the suffering of a man named Job. The book asks profound questions of God's justice, the source of human suffering, and God's overall character. While there is debate into whether or not Job was a real person, the book is held as scripture and is deeply appreciated in Christian and Jewish tradition.

"Mediator"

In the biblical framework, a mediator is someone who stands between God and humanity, reconciling them.

1 Timothy

A book in the New Testament likely written around 63 AD. This book is a letter from the apostle Paul (also called St. Paul) to his dear friend Timothy who is described to be like a son to Paul. This book is one of 2 letters to Timothy.

"Righteousness"

Being right with God, aligned with God. Righteousness typically refers to behavior being aligned with God's instruction, but more holistically refers to general rightstanding with God.

Ecclesiastes

A book in the Old Testament believed to be written by Solomon, though there is some debate about the author. It discusses meaning in life, wisdom, suffering, and life's unpredictability.

Solomon

A son of David, who succeeded as king over Israel after David. Solomon was famous for being wise, wealthy, and building the first temple in Jerusalem.

Romans

A book in the New Testament. Romans is a letter from Paul to the church in Rome. The letter instructs the church, encourages them towards faith in Jesus, and corrects them in certain areas.

Paul

An apostle (one who is sent) of Jesus Christ. Paul was a religious leader who persecuted Christians until his own encounter with Jesus which left him a changed man. After this, he diligently served as a Christian apostle and wrote much of the New Testament in the form of letters.